ALZHEIMER'S
Caring for Your Loved One, Caring for Yourself

ALZHEIMER'S

Caring for Your Loved One

Caring for Yourself

Sharon Fish

SHAW

ALZHEIMER'S
A SHAW BOOK
PUBLISHED BY WATERBROOK PRESS
5446 North Academy Boulevard, Suite 200
Colorado Springs, CO 80918
A division of Random House, Inc.

Unless otherwise indicated, all Scripture quotations are taken from *The Holy Bible: New International Version.* copyright © 1973, 1978, 1984 by the International Bible Society. Used by permission of Zondervan Publishing House. All rights reserved.

Scripture quotations marked RSV are taken from the Revised Standard Version of the Bible, © 1946, 1952, 1971 by the Division of Christian Education of the National Council of Churches of Christ in the USA, and used by permission.

Scripture quotations marked TEV are taken from *Today's English Version (The Good News Bible)*, © 1966, 1971, 1976, 1992 by the american bible Society. Used by permission.

ISBN: 0-87788-014-X

SHAW and its circle of books logo are trademarks of WaterBrook Press, a division of Random House, Inc.

Library of Congress Cataloging-in-Publication Data

Fish, Sharon.
    Alzheimer's : caring for your loved ones, caring for yourself / Sharon Fish.
        p. cm.
    Previously published: Oxford : Lion Pub., 1990.
    Includes bibliographical references and index.
    ISBN 0-87788-014-X
    1. Alzheimer's disease—Patients—Home care. 2. Alzheimer's disease—Patients Family relationships. I. Title.
RC523.2.F57 1996
618.97'6831—dc20   96-1063
                                                                                                                CIP

Printed in the United States of America

02 01 00

10 9 8 7 6 5

To LaVonne Neff,

in memory of our parents

Contents

Acknowledgments

My hope for all who read this book is that you will be encouraged. You are not alone as you reach out to care for your loved ones.

I am deeply grateful to Jack Fisher, Kathleen Fisher Poling, Marian Gierasch, and Mary Butts, four caregivers who formed the Alzheimer's support group in Oneonta, New York, and who faithfully kept the candle burning in monthly meetings for those who needed help and encouragement.

Special thanks to Mary Johnson, who read the original manuscript and shared her heart, and to the dozens of other caregivers who were willing to share their experiences for others, including myself, to learn from. To protect caregivers' privacy, no names are included and, in some instances, certain identifying details have been changed at their request. Scenarios that introduce various chapters weave together all our stories, our fears, our hopes, our feelings. The people described could well be your mother or father, husband or wife, sister or brother, son or daughter.

I would like to thank Dr. Raymond Vickers, M.D., professor in the Department of Family Practice, East Carolina University Medical School, who read and edited the original manuscript with a physician's eye; and also his wife, Barbara, who has given so generously of her time and talents to encourage caregivers for many years in a variety of settings.

Thank you to the following people who lovingly helped me care for my mother: Sylvia Davisson, Pat Gifford, Janet Roseboom, Bunny Rodriquez, Kim Lund, Carol Rose, Katie Jenison, and Debbie Derry. Thanks to the staff at Stamford Nursing Home in Stamford, New York, who cared for my mother as if she were *their* mother during the final days of her life. And thank you to the staff and friends of Inter County Home Care, who were always there when I needed them.

I would also like to acknowledge the special care unit at Kirkhaven, Rochester, New York; Rochester, New York chapter of the Alzheimer's Association; Dr. Eric G. Tangalos, Mayo Clinic Alzheimer's Disease Center, Rochester, Minnesota; and Susan Duncan, Via Christi/St. Francis Regional Medical Center, Wichita, Kansas, for their helpful assistance.

Special thanks to the following for a number of reasons: my original editors at Lion, LaVonne Neff and Bob Bittner, who patiently persisted; Dr. Steven Szebenyi and Dr. Donald Pollock from Bassett Hospital, Cooperstown, New York, who helped me over the years with medical management; Emalene Shepherd of the Writer's Digest School, who watered a vision; and Mary Horner Collins, my current editor at Harold Shaw, who believed this book should remain in print.

My final thanks go to Hazel (Grandma) Brown, Ruth Schweinfurth, Molly Maine, Betty Dean, Cindy Thayer, Dorothy Oswald, and Peggy Turley, who prayed and encouraged, and Madeline Schmitt, nursing professor at the University of Rochester, who patiently waited.

To all I am deeply grateful.

Part One

SOMETHING HAS GONE WRONG

A bruised reed he will not break, and a dimly burning wick he will not quench.

Isaiah 42:3

Chapter 1

Bruised Reeds and Dimly Burning Wicks

Muriel sat down at the kitchen table and slowly buttered her toast. Fifteen minutes of silence, twenty if she was lucky. Quiet time alone to enjoy the toast, a cup of coffee, and a quick read through the morning paper before the real work began: getting her mother up, washed, fed, toileted, walked, and dressed for the day. And then, later in the morning, several loads of laundry including her mother's urine-stained sheets.

"Bye, Mom," Susan hollered as she grabbed her books and headed out the door to catch the waiting school bus.

"Bye," yelled Bruce, scooping up his backpack and racing past his sister.

Muriel glanced out the window and caught a glimpse of the bus as it rounded the curve and disappeared out of sight beyond the hedgerow.

The school year would be over in a few weeks. Unfortunately, Muriel knew the children weren't looking forward to being home all summer. When she'd asked them they said they didn't mind, but her neighbor had told her the truth. When the neighbor had asked Susan how she was going to spend her summer vacation, Susan had just shrugged her shoulders and looked unhappy. And Bruce said, "We ain't goin' no place on account of Grandma."

"Mur. Mur."

Ten of my twenty minutes wasted thinking about something I can't do anything about, Muriel thought.

"Mur. Mur."

"In a minute, Mother," Muriel called back, hastily swallowing the last of the coffee, running her plate under the faucet and shoving it into the dishwasher.

Ruth. Muriel's mother. Ruth was the reason the children weren't looking forward to their summer vacation.

Muriel couldn't blame them. It wasn't easy being thirteen and seven and having a grandparent with Alzheimer's disease living with you twenty-four hours a day. A grandmother who didn't do the things grandmothers were supposed to do—like tell you what adorable grandchildren you were, listen to your stories, and bake you cookies. A grandmother who, instead, sometimes threatened you and didn't even know your name, babbled incoherently at times, and had almost burned your house down trying to boil an egg.

Muriel's father had died fifteen years earlier, and her mother never remarried. Ruth continued to live alone in the old family farmhouse, three miles from Muriel, Carl, and the children. At age sixty-five, Ruth had begun to show signs of memory loss, but the signs were so subtle that Muriel hardly noticed them.

Her mother was forever losing things: her glasses, her checkbook, her keys. When Muriel would drop in unexpectedly she'd often find Ruth rummaging through drawers, muttering under her breath. But then, for as long as Muriel could remember, her mother had misplaced things.

Then her mother stopped remembering.

Birthdays were first. Muriel's. Carl's. Susan's. Bruce's. Her own. Very unlike the mother who had never failed to send a card, buy a present, or bake a cake.

Appointments were next. The podiatrist, hairdresser, dentist—all were forgotten. Muriel had calls from all three of them one month asking where Ruth was.

Muriel's mother had notes posted all over the house. "Memory joggers," Ruth called them. But she still forgot.

And then there were names. Odd, Muriel had thought, that her mother couldn't seem to remember the names of the children one Sunday when she was over for dinner. Ruth kept calling them Sally and Ron, the names of her own sister and brother. The children thought it was a game Grandma was playing. Muriel wasn't so sure.

It was Muriel's husband, Carl, who first realized there was more wrong with Ruth than simple age-related memory loss.

Carl stopped by the farm one morning to get Ruth's grocery list and found his mother-in-law taking a nap in a smoke-filled house. She had put a crumb cake in the oven, turned the oven on high and gone to sleep. The smoke detector was working, but Ruth had removed her hearing aid and, as she told them later, had forgotten where she put it. A look in the kitchen cupboards revealed more black-bottomed pots and pans, ample evidence that cooking was one task Ruth could no longer accomplish safely.

The final straw came several weeks later when Muriel got a phone call. Ruth was at the post office in town, having walked the two miles in the rain. She insisted she was in the bank, wanted to see the balance on her account, and demanded her money. Could Muriel please come and get her mother, asked the postmistress.

Muriel did. She got Ruth, took her home to the farm and started packing.

Relocation hadn't been easy. Ruth became even more confused and disoriented in the new environment. She accused Muriel and Carl of stealing her money and selling the family farm.

The children, then aged ten and four, were a mixed blessing as far as Ruth was concerned. Sometimes she showered them with affection, and they basked in the attention. At other times they were also part of the supposed conspiracy to confiscate her property.

Bruce seemed to go with the flow of Grandma's mood swings, but Susan, who had known the love of a more stable grandmother, had a difficult time accepting the bizarre behavior patterns that emerged. When Ruth had one of her verbal outbursts, Susan would run to her own room and stay there until her mother or father assured her the coast was clear.

Now, three years later, Ruth's paranoia was gone, but Susan's habit of retreat remained. Muriel hoped Susan would outgrow it. And she wished she didn't feel so guilty about the children.

"Mur. Mur," Ruth called from the bedroom, the room Susan had given up when her grandmother moved in.

"Coming, Mother," Muriel called, as she closed the door to the dishwasher and turned it on.

Alzheimer's: A Family Affair

This book is certainly not the first word on Alzheimer's disease, nor will it be the last. Rather it is one voice in a chorus speaking out about a devastating illness affecting the daily lives of millions of people worldwide. People like Muriel and Ruth. People like my mother and your mother, our fathers, husbands, wives, children. The cared for and the caregivers. The loved ones and those who love.

Twenty years of hospital, nursing-home, and home-care experience as a registered nurse have brought me in contact with many caregivers and their loved ones. But my own mother brought the reality of Alzheimer's home. In 1980 she was diagnosed with senile dementia of the Alzheimer's type, and I was able to experience caregiving firsthand for over ten years, from the time I first moved home to help my father cope until her death in a nursing home. In 1989 I decided it was time to write about the things my mother was teaching me and the things I was learning from other caregivers. This book, a revision of the original published in 1990, continues the process of caregiving for me as I share additional experiences from my mother's life, my father's life, and my life.

The scenarios that introduce various chapters in this book are based on the lives of many caregivers I have known. To protect caregivers' privacy, names have been changed and, in some instances, certain identifying details have been altered at their request. But all of the events described actually happened and the people described are real people. In telling their stories I've tried to weave together experiences, reminiscences, and emotions to paint a picture of what Alzheimer's is really like.

This book is primarily for caregivers like myself—those who live with loved ones, visit them in nursing homes and adult homes, or show care and concern from afar. I also wrote this book for caregivers' friends and relations. Without them, caregiving would be a very lonely experience. I hope, too, it will be of value to professional and paraprofessional caregivers who recognize illness as a family affair.

In addition to drawing from my own experience and current research and literature, I interviewed dozens of caregivers who gave me permission to quote them. This gave direction for chapter topics and helped me focus on some primary concerns of caregivers. The inclusion of appendices in this edition was designed with the professional caregiver in mind and for family caregivers needing additional sources of information.

Whenever people talk about Alzheimer's, certain questions come up:

➤ How can I tell if my loved one has Alzheimer's? What are the early signs and symptoms?

➤ What causes Alzheimer's disease? Is it hereditary?

➤ How can I be sure my loved one is getting an accurate diagnosis? What's involved in the diagnostic process?

➤ What are some of the bizarre and bewildering behaviors peculiar to Alzheimer's disease? How can I manage them?

➤ Is there any specific treatment or cure?

➤ What's the purpose for all this suffering? What kind of God would allow this to happen?

➤ How can I meet my own needs as a wife, husband, daughter, son?

➤ Is it normal for me to feel angry, guilty, depressed, or resentful? How can I deal with these emotions?

➤ How can I deal with my loved one's physical needs?

➤ What kinds of resources are available to help care for my loved one at home? How can I pay for this care?

➤ How can a person decide to place a loved one in a nursing home? Is there ever a right time?

➤ Are brain autopsies important? How can I find out about them?

➤ What will death be like for my loved one? What will my loved one's death be like for me?

We will look at each of these questions in detail in later chapters. But first, what is Alzheimer's? Who gets it?

Some Facts about Alzheimer's

Alzheimer's disease is a complex, chronic, progressive, irreversible brain disorder or dementia for which there is no definable cause, no definitive treatment and, to date, no foreseeable cure.

Dementia, the broader diagnostic category of which Alzheimer's disease is a type, is a multifaceted decline of intellectual functions of sufficient severity to interfere with an individual's activities of daily living, career, social relationships, and social activities. Dementia involves personality changes, loss of memory and judgment, and difficulty with abstract thinking and orientation.[1]

The word *dementia* literally means "mind away" or "deprived of mind." Dementing illnesses are the result of one or more disease processes that can drastically alter people's behavior and gradually bankrupt their minds and the lives of entire families. Alzheimer's disease is thought to be the primary cause of incurable dementia for men and women over the age of sixty-five.

In the United States there are over 30 million people older than sixty-five years of age. Of this population, more than 4 million Americans may suffer from Alzheimer's disease. Statistics are similar in other developed countries where life expectancy reaches into the sixties and seventies.

Although Alzheimer's usually occurs after a person reaches the mid-sixties, with a significant increase after age eighty, Alzheimer's can also afflict people in their forties and fifties. It's not just a disease of the old or very old.

The National Institute on Aging projects that Alzheimer's may affect approximately 14 million people in the United States alone within fifty years. The accompanying emotional and economic costs stagger the imagination. While the majority of people with Alzheimer's continue to live in a home environment supported by friends, relatives, and community services, Alzheimer's sufferers currently fill over fifty percent of all nursing-home beds.[2]

The fourth leading cause of death in Americans older than seventy-five, Alzheimer's has been called "the disease of the twentieth century."[3] It may well be the disease of the twenty-first century as well: as the over eighty-five population doubles, one out of every three of us may have an older relative diagnosed with Alzheimer's.

Alzheimer's disease has also been described in the literature and by caregivers as "a funeral that never ends," "a nightmare from which you never wake up," "another name for madness," "the silent epidemic," "the slow death of the mind." One of the most popular and practical books ever written on the subject of Alzheimer's disease is titled *The 36-Hour Day*, reflecting the reality of life for most caregivers.[4] Caring for a loved one with a dementing illness *does* seem to require more than seven days a week, twenty-four hours a day, sixty minutes an hour; the difficulties inherent in caring for someone with Alzheimer's disease are all too real.

But the difficulties are not the whole picture. Caregiving can also be an opportunity for growth. It can make us more patient, more compassionate, and more courageous people. A beautiful passage in the Bible reads, "A bruised reed he will not break, and a dimly burning wick he will not quench" (Isaiah 42:3, RSV). There is hope for the caregiver who feels battered and bruised in the battle against Alzheimer's disease. We need not be broken.

There is also hope for our loved ones. No matter how bizarre or bewildering their behavior, they are still precious people carefully designed in the image and likeness of their Creator. As caregivers, we have daily opportunities to fan the flames of their hearts and spirits as we care for them in love.

And, it is hoped, our own hearts and spirits will be lifted up and comforted in the very process of caregiving as we discover untapped, unrecognized strengths in ourselves and in the people around us.

Chapter 2

Searching for the Truth

"I think my mother has Alzheimer's," a friend confided to me one night. "She has all the symptoms your mother does. She's confused and forgetful. She can't even remember her own name or mine, and she's having a lot of personality changes."

"How long has this been going on?" I asked, puzzled because this was the first time my friend had mentioned her mother's changing behavior.

"Just about a month," she said.

I told my friend her mother's condition might *not* be the more gradually developing disease of Alzheimer's and encouraged her to take her mother to a doctor immediately.

My friend's mother was diagnosed a short time later. She didn't have Alzheimer's. She had a rapidly growing brain tumor.

In past decades, Alzheimer's was one of the most underdiagnosed diseases. Today it has burst out of obscurity to become one of the most overdiagnosed, particularly among friends and family members who have read a lot about it in the popular literature.

Even some health-care professionals are guilty of making the instant diagnosis. Unfortunately, it's still not uncommon to hear caregivers say, "My husband's doctor took one look at him and said, 'He has all the symptoms of Alzheimer's. It's not necessary to run any tests.' "

Yet brain autopsy reports have indicated that some people actually diagnosed with Alzheimer's did not in fact have the disease. They showed none of Alzheimer's characteristic physical changes in the brain, even though they had exhibited symptoms of brain dementia.

(Characteristic physical changes include senile plaques and neurofibrillary tangles that form in the brain tissue of people with Alzheimer's.)[1]

Alzheimer's is not the *only* disease process that causes dementia. Far from it. There are dozens of disorders whose symptoms can mimic those of Alzheimer's disease. While some of these disorders are chronic and incurable, many others can be treated, reversed, or cured completely. Many have nothing to do with the brain at all in relation to cause. Some of these disorders may also coexist with Alzheimer's, exaggerating symptoms.

There is always the need, in the case of memory loss and confusion, to have a complete diagnostic examination as soon as possible. This is true whether the confusion is mild or severe, whatever the person's age. The examination should include a thorough history and physical, various blood tests, a neurological and psychological workup and, in some cases, a psychiatric evaluation.

Diagnosing Alzheimer's is a laborious process of elimination and exclusion. One visit to the doctor will not usually result in a diagnosis. Nor will one test. Diagnosis is difficult. The course of the disease process varies greatly from person to person, and there is always a degree of diagnostic uncertainty.

If you're uncomfortable with the physician your loved one is currently seeing, inquire about physicians in your area who are specialists in geriatric medicine or neurology, experienced in diagnosing and treating dementing illnesses, or willing to make the appropriate referrals. Never feel guilty about seeking a second opinion.

Members of Alzheimer's support groups can be particularly helpful in steering you to sensitive physicians. Your local community or public health nursing agency may also be a good referral source. You'll want a physician you can talk to and trust because you'll probably be seeing a lot of each other.

Evaluating a person for Alzheimer's is not a once-in-a-lifetime experience. Certain tests may need to be repeated at yearly or more frequent intervals as the disease progresses, especially with the younger Alzheimer's sufferer. Early symptoms of Alzheimer's disease are subtle, but if your loved one has Alzheimer's there will be a definite downhill progression. People with Alzheimer's do not get better.

For your own peace of mind and for the health of your loved one, never assume it's Alzheimer's until all the test results are in.

Noticing Changes

Actually, when we think back, Dad started to act depressed after his colostomy surgery in 1968. He felt he was not normal. But then there was more than just the depression. From that point on it seemed all downhill. There were other signs. He was about sixty-four.

As caregivers, *we ourselves* are the single most important diagnostic tool in the search for truth about what's causing our loved one's confusion. Our reflections on the history of his or her behavior changes are invaluable to the physician. Though most physicians will want to question our loved one directly, people in the early stages of Alzheimer's can be masters in the fine art of "cover-up." Not a few physicians have been fooled by the perfectly normal behavior and appearance of people with Alzheimer's in their office. You know things are different at home, but you may need some facts to prove it.

When attempting to reconstruct your loved one's medical and social history, there are two key words to remember: *change* and *onset*. What are the various changes you've noticed in your loved one's life over the past few weeks, months, or years? When did you first notice these changes? Have they been gradual in onset, occurring over a period of time, or have they occurred suddenly?

The time frame for the appearance and progression of symptoms is an important clue for physicians to consider when making a diagnosis and deciding what tests to conduct. Before you go to the hospital or physician's office, think through the following categories. You may even want to write down your answers and take them with you.

Affect and attitude. Has your loved one been unusually anxious, agitated, depressed, apathetic, or withdrawn? When did you first notice these changes? Have there been any major events associated with these changes, such as retirement, relocation, death of a close friend or relative, or surgery?

Behavior. What specific behavior changes have you noticed? Have there been any differences in your loved one's daily routine? Have you noticed any marked personality changes, such as forgetfulness? If so, what exactly is forgotten? How frequently does forgetfulness occur? Has your loved one ever wandered off and gotten lost?

Conversation. Has your loved one experienced any language difficulties? Have there been any problems related to the ability to speak or remember words? Is one word substituted for another at the end of a sentence? Are phrases mixed up or confused? Has speech become slurred or garbled?

Decision making. Have you noticed any changes in decision-making capabilities? Are there any errors in judgment? In relation to what, specifically? Is your loved one having difficulty driving? Is he/she able to do so safely?

Drugs. List any medications being taken, both prescription and over-the-counter. Are medications being taken correctly?

Environment. Are pots and pans burned while cooking? Are there piles of unpaid bills? Is mail stacked up? Is there evidence that your loved one is neglecting nutritional needs?

Family and friends. What have other people—relatives, friends, neighbors, coworkers—noticed about your loved one's behavior?

Grooming and gait disturbances. Is there any change in your loved one's ability to perform various activities of daily living related to personal grooming—bathing, dressing, toileting? Have there been any changes in the ability to walk or maintain their balance?

Habits. What changes have you noticed in your loved one's normal habit patterns? Are there things that are simply too difficult to do now, such as balancing a checkbook, cooking, cleaning, reading, yard work, auto repair, gardening? Are there any favorite hobbies that are no longer engaged in? Have you noticed any changes in the ability and desire to socialize with others?

Illnesses. What specific physical symptoms is your loved one experiencing? Has there been any significant and recent weight loss or weight gain?

Is there a history of any of the following: metabolic disorders such as diabetes or thyroid disease, heart or lung abnormalities, strokes, dizziness, fainting spells, headaches, shaking, seizures? Is there any history of alcoholism?

Has your loved one fallen down or had any past or recent head injuries? Has there been exposure to any toxic chemicals in the workplace? Is there any history of blood transfusions? When and where were they done? Is there any history of Alzheimer's disease or undiagnosed memory loss in your loved one's family? Any familial nervous or mental disease?

As caregivers we need to be sure that no stone has been left unturned in the search for the cause of our loved one's confusion. The stones related to our loved one's history are the ones we need to turn over ourselves.

Maybe It's Not Alzheimer's

In the beginning we said to ourselves, "Dad is just getting old." Even his doctor said so and told us it was probably just hardening of the arteries to the brain. So we thought, well, he's getting old and he's getting senile.

But his confusion wasn't just part of old age, we found out later. We finally took him to a doctor who listened to him, did a good examination and a bunch of tests, and who was willing to tell us more about what was going on.

A good place to start in the search for truth about the cause of our loved one's confusion is with a general physical examination. This will involve more than taking a temperature, pulse, and blood pressure.

Even if the primary dementia is caused by Alzheimer's, there may be associated chronic or acute problems. If these go undiagnosed and untreated, they can make the confusion caused by Alzheimer's worse. On the other hand, some of these conditions may themselves be the cause of the confusion.

Chronic and acute diseases and disabilities. Heart- or lung-related diseases such as congestive heart failure, heart rhythm and valve disorders, pneumonia, and a variety of chronic obstructive lung disorders may contribute to mild or severe oxygen deprivation to the brain. This lack of oxygen, in turn, can cause acute episodes of confusion and can contribute to chronic dementia.

In some cases the culprit of confusion is a chronic cholesterol build-up that results in a narrowing of the arteries supplying blood to the brain. This is called coronary artery disease or atherosclerosis. Coronary artery disease (usually with accompanying hypertension) may, over a period of time, result in a series of small strokes or infarcts in the brain. This can cause an intermittent confusion that is frequently mistaken for Alzheimer's disease and often goes undetected unless the person experiences a massive stroke.

This mini-stroke phenomenon, more frequently seen in men, is called multi-infarct dementia, a type of vascular dementia. It is the second most common cause of confusion in older people, responsible for approximately thirty-five percent of all dementias.[2]

Unlike Alzheimer's, multi-infarct dementia often begins suddenly. Its downhill progression is usually steplike in nature, with plateaus. There may be evidence of specific local or focal neurological impairments such as muscle weakness to an arm or leg or slurred speech, as opposed to the more gradual and generalized global decline of Alzheimer's disease. By supplying the person's history, a caregiver may help the physician distinguish between Alzheimer's and multi-infarct dementia.

People can, and frequently do, suffer from multi-infarct dementia in combination with Alzheimer's. Why is it important to know which problem is causing the person's confusion? Pharmacologic and/or surgical treatments can often eliminate or greatly reduce the likelihood of further stroke activity if the confusion is related to vascular disease rather than the Alzheimer's process. An accurate diagnosis can lead to improved health.

There are also other diseases that may produce progressive dementialike symptoms. The most notable are Binswanger's disease, Huntington's disease, Pick's disease, multiple sclerosis, amyotrophic lateral sclerosis ("Lou Gehrig's disease"), Parkinson's disease, and Creutzfeldt-Jakob disease, an extremely rare brain disorder. An overview of these conditions is included in appendix B.

Sensory impairments or disabilities may also be a factor in confusion. Occasionally when older people appear to be forgetful or confused, they are simply suffering from poor vision and/or hearing loss. Both conditions may be correctable with surgery or mechanical aids.

Deficiencies. The brain needs nutritious food to survive. A poorly nourished brain can contribute to confusion, forgetfulness, irritability, and depression.

People—especially older people who live alone—can suffer from a number of conditions that are diet related. If older people forget to eat, or fail to eat enough of the right kinds of foods, they may wind up with nutritional deficiencies and even chronic malnutrition. Chronic alcoholism can also be a concern. Both conditions are associated with vitamin deficiencies, and some vitamin deficiencies contribute to dementia-like symptoms. If an older person is not drinking enough water, dehydration can also rapidly occur and contribute to lethargy and confusion and sometimes hallucinations.

Depression. Depression and manic depression are two other conditions that mimic Alzheimer's and should always be considered when there is memory loss. Classically depressed people may appear passive, helpless, hopeless, and confused. Behavioral and intellectual responses may be slower than normal. Manic depression may result in mood changes that swing between a state of excitement, or mania, and deep depression.

The onset of depression is usually more rapid than the onset of Alzheimer's and may be triggered by specific events such as the death of a spouse or the loss of a job. There are often accompanying physical signs such as fatigue, insomnia, and loss of weight and appetite.

Current research indicates that twenty to thirty percent of the time, treatable depression accompanies Alzheimer's, exaggerating the symptoms of dementia. Antidepressant medications are often ordered that may help alleviate the symptoms.[3]

Drugs. One of the most commonly overlooked yet correctable causes of confusion in older people is drug toxicity. The effects of many medications extend far beyond the therapeutic purposes for which they were intended. Many have potentially harmful side effects that can include depression, disorientation, and other dementia-like symptoms.

Drug toxicity can result from either a buildup of one specific medication or a combination of drugs that can produce toxic effects, usually over time. It's not unusual for an older person to be taking over a dozen different medications, sometimes prescribed by several different physicians. Some of these drugs can neutralize other drugs when taken together. Or they can do the exact opposite and speed up the absorption of the second drug, often to an overdose level. All drugs, including those we may think of as innocuous over-the-counter pain relievers, cough suppressants, and laxatives, have potential side effects.

Medications have a greater tendency to build up in the bodies of older people because of the decreased filtration rate in the kidneys. Poor circulation, slower general metabolism, constipation, and a lower level of liver detoxification function contribute to drug toxicity as we age.

Medications can also adversely affect the proper absorption of vitamins, minerals, and other nutrients. Overuse of some antacids, for example, can trigger thiamine deficiencies. Medications can also contribute to nutritional and electrolyte imbalances that, in turn, can create confusion. Even something as ordinary as a laxative, if taken indiscriminately, can upset fluid and electrolyte balances.

Older people sometimes consume alcohol in the form of wine or over-the-counter cough medicines or liquid vitamin supplements.

Alcohol does not mix well with many medications. Confusion is a common side effect.

When we take our loved one to the hospital or physician's office, we need to take their medications too, both prescription and over-the-counter, or at least have an accurate record of what they are taking and how long they've been taking it. Medication should definitely be considered as a contributing factor whenever dementia is suspected.

Lab Tests Don't Lie

> I think they did every test imaginable on my husband to make sure he wasn't suffering from something other than Alzheimer's. At forty-five, you want to make sure.

No examination for Alzheimer's would be complete without blood work and other laboratory tests. All of them help to rule out other possible causes of dementia. While not every test will be used by every physician on every person showing symptoms of dementia, some of these certainly will be performed.

Blood tests. A complete blood count (CBC) should be done to rule out the possibility of any underlying acute or chronic infectious process that can cause symptoms similar to Alzheimer's. The CBC can also detect other conditions such as blood cancers or anemia. Low hemoglobin and hematocrit levels can contribute to confusion when there are not enough red blood cells carrying oxygen to the brain.

More specific blood chemistries can measure folic acid and vitamin B-12 levels. Low vitamin B-12 levels may be associated with pernicious anemia. Symptoms are depression and irritability. Low B-12 and folate levels also produce dementia-like symptoms.

Diabetes and other metabolic or endocrine disorders can contribute to marked irritability, personality changes, and confusion. They can be detected by blood-chemistry tests if suspected.

Abnormally high or low doses of thyroid hormone can trigger dementia-like symptoms and can be detected through various thyroid hormone level studies. Abnormally high levels of circulating calcium and sodium, and low sodium levels with accompanying electrolyte imbalances, can also trigger symptoms of dementia.

Poisoning with certain metals such as aluminum, manganese, lead, or mercury has been implicated in dementia, as have pesticides, carbon monoxide, and industrial pollutants. Blood levels can be tested for many of these.

In the nineteenth century, the number one cause of confusion was thought to be syphilis. While it is not generally a major cause of dementia today, a complete work-up for dementia may include a blood test for chronic venereal disease.

Acquired immune deficiency syndrome (AIDS) is another infectious process that can't be automatically ruled out. Dementia is a frequent complication of AIDS. Blood studies to detect the presence of the human immunodeficiency virus (HIV) may be done *if* the symptoms and health history indicate a need.

Urine tests. Urine testing can rule out an acute urinary tract infection that, in the elderly, may cause confusion. High sugar and acetone readings in the urine can also indicate diabetes and the need for more extensive blood work. Urine and blood tests may also reveal evidence of medication overdose.

Spinal fluid tests. The spinal column is part of the central nervous system. The cerebral spinal fluid that courses through the spinal column also bathes the brain.

Spinal taps, or lumbar punctures (LPs), are recommended by some physicians as a diagnostic tool if there is a reason to suspect they would help rule out an infectious process. In this procedure, a small amount of spinal fluid is withdrawn from the spinal column, then analyzed.

Brain tumors, some blood-vessel diseases, and acute and chronic infectious processes such as meningitis and tuberculosis may be diagnosed through spinal taps.

The Mind Matters

When my mother was initially diagnosed with senile dementia of the Alzheimer's type, I went into the examining room with her when she saw the neurologist. I can still remember the "conversation" my mother had with the young neurology resident.

"I just want to ask you a few questions," the resident began.

"Okay," my mother replied.

"What year is it?" he asked.

"1960," she said.

"No, it's 1980," he corrected her. "What month is it?"

"May," she said.

"No, it's December," he said. "What date is it now?"

"The first. Is that right?" my mother asked.

"No, it's the tenth," he told her. "What is the day of the week?"

"You're so smart, you tell me," said Mom.

That concluded the mental-status exam.

What year is it now? What month is it? What date? What day of the week? For most of us, answers to these questions trip off our tongues without much thought. But for someone with a progressive memory loss like Alzheimer's, even the simplest questions can draw a blank.

> The doctor never actually saw my father's bizarre behavior. He wondered if it was my mother's imagination. Until he could see the problems for himself, he wouldn't believe her.
>
> The doctor finally took Dad into a room and asked him some questions. Dad didn't know if he was married. He didn't know his religion. He didn't know who the president was. He didn't know the month or the day or the season.
>
> The doctor finally realized my mother had been telling the truth.

A neurologist and/or your loved one's own general physician may do a mental-status or mini-mental status exam. The various tests that are part of the exam indicate the ability of different parts of the brain to function. The more complex questions can give clues to the cause and progression of the dementia.[4]

Mental-status exams generally measure what is known as cognitive functioning. The word *cognition*, used extensively by health-care professionals when talking about the dementias, means "the process or quality of knowing." Cognition includes our ability to reason and remember, perceive and make judgments, conceive and imagine—all those mental activities that make us uniquely human, uniquely us.

Mental-status exams may be repeated over time to better assess our loved one's level of functioning and rate of change. The questions used test a number of different areas as follows.

Degree of orientation to time, place, person, and object. Do they know what day it is, where they are, who they are? Are they aware of current events? For example, do they know who the president is? Do they know their phone number and their address? If shown familiar objects such as a pencil or a watch, can they name them?

Memory for remote and recent past. Can they tell when and where they were born? Do they know the names of their parents? Can they repeat from memory a simple series of numbers or familiar objects, five minutes after they are told what those numbers or objects are?

Mathematical skills. Can they solve simple math calculations? For example, can they count backward from one hundred in multiples of three or four?

Abstract reasoning ability and judgment. Do they know the meaning of simple proverbs such as "A bird in the hand is worth two in the bush"? If they were told their stove was on fire in their kitchen, what would they do? Is their response logical?

Reading, writing, and symbolic drawing skills. Are they able to read? Do they understand what they are reading? Are they able to construct a sentence or a paragraph? Can they copy a simple design such as two overlapping triangles or rectangles? Can they draw the face of a clock and write the appropriate numbers in the right places?

We often take our minds for granted. The mental-status exam reminds us of how much they really do matter and of how they can be adversely affected by a disease such as Alzheimer's.

Having Your Head Examined

We're all familiar with the phrase "You ought to have your head examined." This, in fact, may be just what the doctor orders for a confused person who might be suffering from Alzheimer's disease. When my mother began having symptoms of memory loss, the last thing she wanted to do was to go to a physician. "I don't trust them," she'd say when my father and I encouraged her to visit a nearby medical center.

I finally made an appointment with the nurse practitioner in our small town. I thought the fact that she was a woman might help make my mother feel more at ease, and I thought the small office would seem less imposing than a big hospital.

I was wrong on both counts.

My mother reluctantly agreed to the appointment, but we hadn't been in the waiting room more than five minutes when she headed out the door at top speed. "I'm all right," she insisted. "All right."

One day, after several more episodes like this, I got a call at work from the town grocer. Mom had been downtown making her usual morning rounds from post office to coffee shop to grocery store. The grocer had noticed my mother seemed more confused than usual. "The side of her mouth is drooping a bit," he said. "She's unsteady on her feet, but she keeps insisting she's okay and won't let me call an ambulance."

I got in my car and drove the eight miles home in about five minutes. There was my mother coming out of the bank, leaning to the left. I knew the signs. She looked as if she'd had a small stroke.

"Get in the car, Mom," I said.

"No."

"Mom, please get in the car."

"No," she insisted.

Thankfully, my mother was small. I got out and maneuvered her into the car, fastened her seat belt, and drove to the hospital. She protested all the way but calmed down as we neared the emergency entrance.

When we got there, I was able to speak to a physician I knew. He seized the opportunity to admit her and then give her a brain, or

CT, scan. A short time later, she was officially diagnosed as having Alzheimer's. There was no evidence on the scan of any past stroke activity.

Another caregiver shared with me his initial experience with the diagnostic process.

> My wife had been going to one hospital for her eyes. Laser treatments. And one day her doctor said, "You know, it wouldn't hurt your wife to have an MRI scan done." I asked why.
>
> He said, "Well, in talking to her there are times when she doesn't answer me."
>
> I said to him, "I know that. I thought she was just ignoring me."
>
> "No," he said. "It's much more than that."

A thorough neurological examination for mental impairment may include an EEG, CT, or MRI scan either early in the investigative process or after more simple tests have been done without a diagnosis being made.[5] The *EEG*, or electroencephalogram, measures electrical activity in the brain. It involves attaching tiny wires called electrodes to the side of the head with a pastelike substance. The brain waves of people with Alzheimer's may appear perfectly normal, or they may show abnormally slow electrical activity.

EEGs can help identify other causes of dementia with symptoms that mimic Alzheimer's, such as delirium and various seizure disorders, like epilepsy, that may have gone undiagnosed or been misdiagnosed in the past.

A *CT* scan, or computed tomography, is a computer-drawn x-ray of the brain itself, and is the most frequently used imaging technique.

Normally we all experience a certain degree of brain atrophy or shrinkage and brain-weight loss as we get older, due to a decreased number of living brain cells. Alzheimer's disease speeds up the process of cellular shrinkage and cellular death significantly.

CT scans can measure brain atrophy by indicating space between the skull and the brain related to widespread loss of nerve tissue in the cerebral cortex, or outer covering of the brain. A diagnosis of mild to severe atrophy can be made, depending on the size of the space. Usually, but not always, the greater the degree of dementia, the greater the atrophy.

Inner spaces of the brain, or ventricles, where cerebro-spinal fluid normally circulates, also increase in size as brain substance decays and is replaced by more fluid. The size of the ventricles may be directly proportional to the degree of dementia.

Magnetic resonance imaging, known as *MRI* or *NMR*, is a more recently developed head-examining technique. MRI provides a more detailed picture of the brain than does a CT scan, and may be ordered if CT scan results are judged insufficient to make a diagnosis.

Unfortunately, the CT scan or MRI alone can't provide an absolute diagnosis of Alzheimer's disease. Brain shrinkage is not always apparent. In any case, the only absolute proof is found through brain autopsy following death. But what these tests *can* do, in conjunction with other tests, is eliminate other possible causes of dementia. Scans can detect brain tumors, cysts, blood clots, or subdural hematomas that may have resulted from falls and blows to the head; normal-pressure hydrocephalus, or an excess of fluid on the brain related to head injury, meningitis, or encephalitis; and the stroke activity of multi-infarct dementia.

Pick's disease, a dementia producing lesser degrees of memory loss than Alzheimer's but greater degrees of socially and sexually inappropriate behavior, may also be detected. It is evidenced by severe atrophy in the area of the temporal cortex of the brain. Again, this diagnosis is not conclusive apart from brain autopsy.

In addition to EEGs and CT and MRI scans, *PET* (positron emission tomography) procedures are sometimes done in research facilities that complement rather than replace the more common types of structural imaging methods.

In the PET procedure, radioactive glucose is injected into the brain and studies are done to determine what areas of the brain are able to metabolize the glucose. If someone suffers from Alzheimer's, it is anticipated that there will be certain "dead" areas in the brain, most notably in the temporal and parietal lobes, where no metabolism will take place.

An even more recent diagnostic tool is called *SPECT* (single photon emission computed tomography). This is a procedure researchers hope will help separate treatable types of dementia from irreversible types such as Alzheimer's.

EEGs, CT and MRI scans, and PET and SPECT procedures are not painful, but they may be frightening to a person who's confused to begin with. They are usually done in busy hospitals on stretchers or tables that are cold, hard, and uncomfortable. If a person fails to relax or is moving around, it may be difficult to get accurate test results. Mild sedation may be ordered prior to the test.

One caregiver told his spouse he was taking her to the beauty parlor. When she arrived at the hospital, she was delighted. The bowl-shaped CT scanner looked like a giant hair dryer. Once her head was in place, she promptly fell asleep.

Reassurance, going with your loved one to the exam area (something you may have to insist on), and appealing to your loved one's sense of humor may all be necessary.

If a person's symptoms are of recent onset, one or more of the foregoing procedures may be done. If symptoms have advanced and progressed for several years, they may not be. But they are all options to consider when you and your loved one's physician are searching for the truth.

Chapter 3

Facing the Facts

Every day at 11:00 A.M. the taxi pulls up in front of the townhouse on 71st and Vine. The driver toots, turns off the engine, lights a cigarette and waits for Ralph Murphy, who will soon appear with an umbrella in one hand, shopping bag in the other, and an overcoat thrown over his shoulder. Ralph will suddenly disappear again because he's forgotten to feed the cat, check the burners on the stove, or turn out the lights. But he's seventy-five and entitled to a little memory lapse, thinks the cab driver.

"Hi ya, Jack."

"Hi ya, Mr. Murphy. The usual, right?"

"Right, Jack. Same time. Same station. Every day. You know me. Can't keep a good man down."

The taxi inches its way along 71st, turns down Chestnut and then onto River, and finally stops in front of a two-story brick building surrounded by azaleas. The sign on the door reads, "Riverview Manor Convalescent Home."

"See you at 2:30," says Ralph Murphy, handing Jack a ten-dollar bill.

"I'll be here," says the driver. "Say hello to Mrs. Murphy for me."

"Will do, Jack. Will do."

Inside, he calls out, "Honey. Honey, I'm here. It's your Ralph."

Harriet Murphy doesn't turn to acknowledge her husband. Instead, she's looking out her window, pointing with her finger in the general direction of the parking lot across the street.

"What are you looking at, Honey?"

Harriet doesn't respond. She just continues to point.

"It's about time for dinner. Are you ready, Honey?" asks Ralph.

"Hungry," says Harriet, looking at her husband for the first time. "That's my girl."

Ralph lays his coat and umbrella on the bed, puts his shopping bag in Harriet's lap, grips the handles of her wheelchair, and propels it out the door. They head for the dining room of the nursing home where one tray waits for Harriet and another waits for him, courtesy of the management. Ralph feeds Harriet her dinner and then eats his own, as he has every day for the past four years.

After dinner they go out on the patio and look at the birds around the bird feeder and Ralph talks to Harriet. He tells her stories about the kids and grandkids and great grandkids, and they look at all the pictures he keeps in the shopping bag.

Then Ralph wheels Harriet back to her room. He kisses her good-bye, tells her he loves her, goes out to the desk, jokes with the nurses for a few minutes, heads for the lobby, gets in his waiting taxi and leaves.

"How'd it go today, Mr. Murphy?" asks Jack.

"Not so good, not so good."

Jack doesn't say anything more. He knows that today Ralph Murphy just wants to sit back and remember.

It's been a long time since that day in June. Over fifteen years. But Ralph still remembers it as if it were yesterday. You don't forget a thing like that. It's not every day your wife accuses you of being a rapist.

They'd stopped at that little motel in Virginia. The Forget-Me-Not, they called it. The name seemed appropriate. Ralph had gone out to get them a couple of sandwiches and coffee. When he came back to the motel, there they were. The police. Ten men with guns that looked like cannons and five cars with lights revolving round and round. Sirens blowing.

So much for a quiet evening in Virginia, he remembers thinking. Maybe this wasn't such a good choice of a motel. Cheap. But . . .

Then, before he could open his car door, someone opened it for him, pulled him out, threw him against the fender, told him to get his hands in the air and started searching him.

"Are you the man who claims to be Ralph Murphy?"

"I am Ralph Murphy," he said. "What's the matter?"

"We've had a complaint from the woman in Room 22. She claims you're holding her against her will."

"Room 22? That's my wife!"

"That's what you say. She says different."

"What do you mean?"

"I mean she called the operator, asked for the police, and said you kidnapped her, raped her, and are holding her in that room."

At that point Ralph started laughing.

"What's so funny?"

"She's my wife," Ralph repeated. "My wife. She gets very confused sometimes. Haven't you talked to her?"

"Yes, we did," said the policeman. "And you're right. She did seem confused. She told us it was 1931 and a few other things that didn't make much sense. I guess maybe you're right. You act like you're her husband, but you're still going to have to prove it. Is there someone we can call?"

"My son. In Florida. That's where we were headed."

So they went to the motel office where Ralph gave the police the number and they placed the call. His son verified that Ralph was indeed his father, that Harriet was his mother and that, yes, she had been having some memory problems.

"If you've got any more overnight stops to make, Mr. Murphy," said the policeman, "you might want to cancel your trip. Either that or don't let your wife out of your sight. We believed you. The next time you might not be so lucky. "

The next morning, Ralph and Harriet Murphy headed back to Pennsylvania.

The following week, Ralph made an appointment at the medical center. When he came out of the doctor's office two weeks later with a tentative diagnosis of Alzheimer's disease, he knew there'd be no more trips to Florida. He couldn't deny the decline any longer.

The next few years were hell on earth for him. Harriet's suspicions grew worse. She continued accusing him of molesting her. "I don't know you. Get out!" she'd scream at him if he tried to come into their bedroom.

He tried to tell Harriet she had an illness when she asked, as she often did, what was wrong with her. "You have an illness of your mind," he'd say. Then she'd get upset and accuse *him* of being crazy.

Then there was the night she ran away. Luckily he was a light sleeper. He got up and stumbled downstairs when he realized she was gone. He headed for the bridge. And sure enough, there was Harriet getting ready to jump off the bridge.

This time Ralph was grateful to see the police who were patrolling the area. They helped him get her into the car and take her home.

"You know, you're going to need some help with her," one of the policemen said.

"I know," he said.

Three weeks later, Harriet was admitted to Riverview Manor. She hated the place at first. She accused the nursing assistants, the housekeeping staff, even the nursing-home administrator of molesting her, of holding her against her will. And Ralph knew she talked to them about him. What a terrible person he'd been to her. How unfeeling he was for "dumping her off" like this.

But Harriet was safe. She was clean, dry, and fed. She was well taken care of. For that, he was grateful.

"Same time tomorrow, Mr. Murphy?" asks the cabby, pulling up in front of the townhouse.

"Same time, same station. Thanks, Jack."

Ralph Murphy gets out of the cab, pays the driver, waves, and starts up the steps. When he reaches the top step he pauses, turns around, and doubles back to the waiting taxi. He's forgotten his overcoat.

Blowing Away the Myths

"In short, I believe that the major diseases of human beings have become approachable biological puzzles, ultimately solvable. . . . Strokes and senile dementia, and cancer, and arthritis are not natural aspects of the human condition, and we ought to rid ourselves of such impediments as quickly as we can," wrote Dr. Lewis Thomas.[1]

In addition to chronic and dementing diseases, another impediment we need to rid ourselves of is myths.

In relation to dementia in general and Alzheimer's in particular, myths abound. There's a lot of fiction mixed in with the facts, largely arising out of fear and/or lack of knowledge.

Myth Number 1: All old people get senile.

All confused people age, but all people who age do not become confused. Chronology is not synonymous with confusion.

In actual fact, only about five percent of all people over the age of sixty-five are severely impaired intellectually due to dementia. An additional ten percent may be mildly to moderately impaired. That leaves eighty-five percent of people over sixty-five with minds that, intellectually speaking, function very well indeed.

Any sign of forgetfulness in our loved ones or even ourselves should not trigger a panic attack. Just because you forgot where you put your car keys, missed an appointment with your dentist, or can't remember where you stored last summer's picnic supplies does not mean you're in the early stages of Alzheimer's. Isolated instances of forgetfulness may simply be related to information overload or the natural memory loss we all experience from time to time.

As we grow up we grow old, and our brains are included in this aging process. Any one of us, if we live into our seventies, eighties, or nineties, will undoubtedly experience a small degree of forgetfulness. That's because the senile plaques and neurofibrillary tangles that are so characteristic of Alzheimer's are also present in normal aging brains. But, unlike the plaques and tangles of Alzheimer's, they are scattered throughout the brain and are fewer in number. Although they can contribute to occasional memory lapses, especially when we're under stress, they don't result in full blown dementia for most of us.[2]

Myth Number 2: If you keep your mind active and read more books, you won't get Alzheimer's.

Neither Alzheimer's disease nor any of the other incurable dementias can be prevented or staved off by keeping your mind active.

Alzheimer's is no respecter of persons. It knows no social, sexual, ethnic, occupational, or educational boundaries.

Myth Number 3: Alzheimer's disease is contagious.

Alzheimer's is *not* contagious. You can't catch it like you can AIDS or the flu. It's not bloodborne or airborne; it is related to a specific disease process.

Myth Number 4 : The confusion could easily be cleared up if the blood flowed better. I've heard there are pills you can take that dilate the blood vessels.

Some drugs, called *vasodilators*, increase the diameter of the blood vessels in the brain. Alzheimer's, however, is not a vascular disease, and many physicians believe that vasodilators can in fact be harmful to elderly people with Alzheimer's-type dementia. Vasodilators also dilate peripheral blood vessels in the arms and legs and can actually reduce the pressure available for adequate cerebral blood flow. Decreased blood pressure, such as that which frequently occurs when a person suddenly stands up, can result in lightheadedness and falls, especially in Alzheimer's victims who have difficulty maintaining balance and coordination. If used at all, vasodilators should be used with caution and carefully evaluated by both physician and caregiver.

Myth Number 5: There are many treatments for Alzheimer's disease.

To date, there are no recommended treatments for Alzheimer's disease. There *are*, however, many false prophets in the world eager to take our hard-earned money. They advocate any number of cures and correctives and sometimes even try to pinpoint a cause. Their bogus remedies range from massive doses of megavitamins, to chelation therapy designed to rid the body of excess aluminum. Others offered the so-called seaweed cure of blue-green algae that was widely advertised and marketed before finally being pulled off the market by the Food and Drug Administration due to its potentially dangerous and unadvertized side effects.

When we see our loved one deteriorating before our eyes, it's only natural to want to grasp at any available straw if there's even a remote possibility it might help alleviate some of the symptoms of Alzheimer's and slow the disease process. But it's also natural and in our best interests to ask questions before investing our money for something that, in the long run, could make our loved one's condition worse.

When in doubt about an advertised home remedy or an expensive treatment offered in some out-of-the-way place, the best thing to do is nothing—until you have called or written the Alzheimer's Association and requested information. They can also give you information about legitimate experimental drug trials being conducted with Alzheimer's sufferers. There are many in progress. Additional information about medications used to treat Alzheimer's is included in appendix C.

The Aluminum Question

Many myths and misconceptions currently revolve around the aluminum question. Information has appeared in the popular media that has frightened many people into throwing out anything in the house that was aluminum-based, thinking they could prevent or slow the progression of dementia by eliminating aluminum from their lives.

Aluminum is the third most common element in the universe. We're all exposed to it daily in the food we eat, the water we drink, the medications we take, the deodorants we use. Aluminum is everywhere. Some people also experience occupational exposure to dust containing aluminum or aluminum compounds.

Although it has been known for some time that higher-than-normal concentrations of aluminum salts have been found in the brain cells of people who suffered from Alzheimer's and other dementias, most researchers believe that excess aluminum is the *result*, not the cause, of the disease process.

There is, however, a growing body of circumstantial evidence linking aluminum with Alzheimer's disease. Aluminum is one of the few substances known to cause memory loss and brain tangles when injected into certain animals. The tangles are similar, though not identical, to those which occur in humans. Aluminum has also been implicated in "dialysis dementia." When the aluminum was removed from the dialysis fluid of some patients with kidney disease, the dementia they had been experiencing also reversed.

None of this is proof that aluminum contributes to the degenerative changes which cause Alzheimer's disease. However, it may be that some people are more at risk because of genetic or other factors and would benefit from a reduction in their intake of and exposure to aluminum. For the present, you may feel it is prudent to avoid foods containing aluminum additives and to use nonaluminum pans and utensils, particularly for cooking acidic foods which are known to leech more aluminum from the pan.

Further research is needed before any definite conclusions can be drawn. It is helpful to remember that even if a clear link is found with Alzheimer's, the risk from any past or present exposure to aluminum is still small. Iron, zinc, and mercury are three other elements currently under investigation by researchers.[3]

There is, at present, no treatment or cure for Alzheimer's disease. But there is hope. Alzheimer's is not a normal process of aging. It is a disease, a deviation from the norm. And, as we've learned through experience over the years, all diseases *are* solvable biological puzzles that may one day reveal to us the reasons for their existence.

For the sake of our loved ones and for future generations, we need to pray that day will come soon.

Don't Deny the Decline

> My aunt became very frustrated. She knew there was something desperately wrong with her, and she would sit in her chair and whimper a lot. She always had this sad, sad look. And she thought—and we thought—she was losing her mind.

There were other things, as I look back, that I should have noticed about my wife. In November of 1976 she wanted to have our wills made out. She kept insisting. I wonder if she knew something then I didn't know or even suspect?

"What's the use?" I remember my husband saying to me when he first started to lose his memory. "What's the point of living?"

People in the early stages of Alzheimer's disease need all the support they can get from family, friends, relatives, and the health-care community. They need to be assured they aren't going crazy, that life is not over for them, that they are still loved and accepted.

Denial is a very common reaction to the diagnosis of Alzheimer's and to the initial symptoms of memory loss, even before a diagnosis is made.

We may deny because our loved one's behavior doesn't fit our expectations of a disease. Most people are used to equating illness with observable signs. People with Alzheimer's usually look healthy and alert. They may, in fact, have considerably more energy than we do. Instead of blaming a disease, we attribute their confusion to the myth of senility, or to various changes that occur in mid to late life.

I didn't realize there was anything wrong with my husband for a very long time. He was always so healthy and still is, even though he's been diagnosed with Alzheimer's for over four years. In the beginning I just thought his memory problems were part of his aging, and I guess I thought that if your mind was slipping badly your body should be falling apart too. His wasn't.

My mother was always a little eccentric and a bit of a loner. She just seemed to get more eccentric as the years progressed.

> She withdrew from life more and more after she retired. But she looked so healthy we didn't worry about it.

> Actually we thought Mom was going through menopause. She seemed to have all the signs and symptoms, though they were a bit exaggerated.

We may also deny out of shame or embarrassment. In past generations, families with relatives who were mentally ill or mentally retarded kept them "in the closet," so to speak. They never talked about them outside the immediate family. And, in some cases, people *literally* kept their relatives in the closet.

For some families, there's still a stigma attached to mental illness and mental retardation. This stigma can carry over into the way we feel about a loved one with dementia.

We may also think people outside our immediate family won't understand our loved one's bizarre behavior and will judge us. We're sure they're saying, "There's Harry again, acting strange. Why doesn't Virginia *do* something?"

So, embarrassed by our loved one's behavior, we try to protect everyone involved from potentially embarrassing situations.

> In the beginning we didn't know what was happening to Dad. When he started acting strange in front of other people, we were embarrassed. We tried to cover it up because of our embarrassment. Actually we ourselves were immature.

> My wife would make a fool of herself in restaurants. She'd say suggestive things to the waiters and waitresses. One time she even pinched a waiter on the rear. I was embarrassed to death and apologized for her behavior. Then, finally, I stopped taking her places altogether.

We may deny because the truth is too painful to accept.

> My daughter will sit next to her mother for hours at a time now and her mother won't speak to her, won't recognize her. I know it's hard on her. Awful hard. My daughter didn't want to accept her mother's sickness in the first place.
>
> The doctor told her, "You've got to start accepting it. You've got to tell your children what's going on. It's not going to get better."
>
> And the doctor was right. It didn't.

There's also a natural tendency for us to want to preserve the lives and livelihoods of our loved ones for as long as possible.

> I wrote my husband's cover letters for him when he was applying for jobs. I knew it was stupid. He wouldn't have been able to do any of those jobs anyway. But I didn't want to see him give up. It was denial, I guess. Either that or blind faith.

> There was a lot of denial on my part. I didn't want things to end. I didn't want him not to be able to drive anymore. His self-esteem was so shaken anyway that I just wanted him to do what he could for as long as possible. So I let him drive, even when I knew he wasn't safe on the road. And I prayed a lot.

It's very easy for us as caregivers to deny because our loved ones deny as well. They can make tremendous efforts to compensate for their failing faculties.

> I'm sure my husband had Alzheimer's for several years before he was diagnosed. But he was always so good at concealing his memory loss. He joked about it a lot, about how when he got older he just had so many more things to think

about that it was easy to have more things to forget. I thought that made sense.

Sometimes the health-care community doesn't help our situation and, at times, can even make it worse. Physicians aren't immune to the myth of senility.

> For three years my husband told the doctors he was having trouble with his memory. For three years the doctors kept telling him, "Everybody does when they get to a certain age." When things got so bad my husband couldn't perform his job, they finally started to listen.

In the case of Alzheimer's, we might sometimes feel as if we'd rather not know. But ignorance is not really bliss. To be forewarned is to be forearmed. There are six good reasons why, sooner or later, we have to stop denying.

Six Reasons to Face the Facts

1. Information drives away fear.

Early recognition of Alzheimer's disease can help us deal with our own fears more realistically. One reason Alzheimer's is so frightening is that it makes us feel out of control. We can't prevent it, arrest it, or stop it. One of the best ways to allay this fear is through knowledge and understanding of the disease itself. There are many reputable sources from which we can get reliable information. The more information we have to draw from, the better able we'll be to cope with this devastating disease.

One of the best sources of reliable information is the Alzheimer's Association, formerly known as the Alzheimer's Disease and Related Disorders Association (ADRDA). Since its founding in 1980, the Association has grown from a group of twelve volunteers to a nationwide network of hundreds of regional chapters and local support groups. There are Alzheimer's Associations in over twenty countries.

The Alzheimer's Association has several purposes:

➤ It supports research into the causes and possible cures for Alzheimer's disease and other forms of dementia.

➤ It helps organize caregiver support groups in communities around the world to assist, encourage, and educate caregivers.

➤ It sponsors educational programs and provides written and audiovisual information on Alzheimer's disease and related disorders for both professional and nonprofessional caregivers.

➤ It advocates for caregivers and people with Alzheimer's disease in areas of legislation—locally, nationally, and internationally.

The earlier we are aware of information and available resources, the less likely we are to be faced with a full-blown crisis later, when management problems become increasingly difficult and we need outside help.

2. Our loved ones must be kept safe.
Denial can become dangerous—especially for the loved one living alone, as many people do in the early stages of Alzheimer's. If our loved one is in danger of falling, of setting the house on fire because of forgetfulness, or of wandering off and getting lost, the time has come to actively intervene, whether we want to or not. Independence is not something that can be preserved indefinitely for someone with Alzheimer's.

This recognition of danger may not mean suddenly uprooting loved ones and moving them in with us, but it will mean providing for their safety in practical ways, such as hiring home-care workers or a live-in companion.

3. Our loved ones may benefit from ongoing research.
To date, there are no marketable drugs that claim to treat Alzheimer's, but many caregivers credit experimental drug trials with

alleviating some of the symptoms of the disease. Drug trials are being conducted all over the world at various hospitals and research centers. The earlier the diagnosis, the greater the chance an Alzheimer's sufferer will qualify for a program should he or she wish to do so. Local or regional support groups or chapters can help identify various locations where studies are going on. The Alzheimer's Association can also provide information.

4. The entire family should play a role in caregiving.

Alzheimer's disease is a family affair. In most instances, spouses, siblings, children, grandchildren, great-grandchildren, and an assortment of in-laws are involved. All have roles and responsibilities when it comes to caregiving, and open communication early in the course of the disease is important to ensure that the burden of caregiving is shared.

5. Financial arrangements must be made.

Alzheimer's not only bankrupts the mind; it can also take its toll on family finances and savings accounts. Insurance coverage rarely pays for chronic custodial care, yet this is the type of care we'll eventually need whether our loved one stays at home or is placed in a nursing home. Home care isn't cheap, and the prospects of nursing-home placement—with astronomical costs that continue to rise—can create panic. The best advice for caregivers is to consult a lawyer familiar with the legalities governing estates and the care of older people in varying situations. Caregivers need to consider obtaining a durable power of attorney enabling them to take charge of their loved one's affairs when it becomes necessary to do so.

The book *Understanding Alzheimer's Disease*, published by the Alzheimer's Association, features several excellent chapters devoted to legal and financial issues.[4] The Alzheimer's Association can also steer caregivers to other resources that are relevant to specific situations. They publish a newsletter that is an excellent source of up-to-date information for family and professional caregivers.

6. The future must be planned.

An early diagnosis of Alzheimer's can give both you and your loved one time to think together about what you would do if you had a future with many long years ahead of you. Then, think about living out the future *now*. For example, you may want to take early retirement or go on that trip you've been putting off.

Memory loss in the early stages of Alzheimer's does not mean people are incapable of making any rational decisions. On the contrary, they need to be involved in planning their own future to as great a degree as possible. This may even include the difficult decision of whether or not they want to be resuscitated should they have a cardiac or respiratory arrest in the final stages of their illness.

Alzheimer's is a fatal disease. It's been called a terminal illness that results in a slow death of the mind. As with any terminal illness, it is a natural initial reaction to deny. Our denial of Alzheimer's disease acts as a cushion. It softens the blow to protect us early on from the emotional pain and distress we might otherwise not be able to handle. Yet to finally admit that our loved ones are experiencing more than "just a little memory loss" can be a relief. For them and for us.

One caregiver I interviewed told me about an experience of her young son. They were at a family picnic at a public beach near a group of people who suffered from mild to severe mental and physical disabilities.

"A lot of the other children seemed afraid of them," said the caregiver. "Their behavior was a bit different, and many of the children seemed to be intentionally avoiding them. They'd back away. But not my son. He said, 'Look, Mommy. There are some sick people from the hospital.'

"My son certainly wasn't afraid of them. He walked right up to their group, reached out, shook some of their hands and introduced himself. I think it had a lot to do with him spending so much time with his grandmother who has Alzheimer's. He's used to being around people whose behavior is different."

We can learn a lot from this young child. As caregivers we need to have the courage to walk up to the disease, look it squarely in the eye, and shake it by the hand. We need to say, "I am not afraid of you, and I'm not going to deny your existence." And we need to say to our loved one, "I love you. I'm not ashamed of your behavior. We'll fight this disease together." It's this kind of realistic and healthy attitude that can carry us beyond the inevitable denial and move us into acceptance.

Note: If you are a caregiver, write the Alzheimer's Association and request an order form of available information. If you don't belong to a chapter or support group that gets the Association's regular newsletter, ask to be put on their mailing list. The national headquarters can also refer you to an Alzheimer's chapter near you and provide additional information on various issues.

The national headquarters' address is:

Alzheimer's Association
919 North Michigan Avenue
Suite 1000
Chicago, Illinois 60611-1676

Their toll-free information number is:

1-800-292-3900

In addition to information that can be ordered through the Alzheimer's Association, there are many other resources available. A number of them are listed in appendix A of this book.

Chapter 4

What's Happening Upstairs?

Well, here they were again. Four o'clock on a Friday afternoon and headed for the truck-stop diner. Precisely at three, Anna had started pacing up and down, up and down in the kitchen at home, repeating the same old question, "When are we going? When are we going? When are we going to go?" The same question she'd asked nearly every afternoon for the past six months.

Sam couldn't understand it.

His daughter had tried to explain it to him. "It's part of her disease, Dad. She can't help it. People with Alzheimer's often repeat themselves, over and over again."

Darnedest disease he'd ever seen. Why couldn't she have gotten sugar diabetes or broken her hip? That you could live with. But no, Anna had to go and get senile.

Funny thing about it was she'd always been so smart. Always had her head in a book. Did the taxes. Kept the checkbook. Paid the bills.

Now Sam had to do all those things. All those things he didn't like. He'd never had a head for figures. Anna was the brains of the outfit.

He sure didn't expect retirement to be like this. They were supposed to be able to relax and enjoy life after forty years of working in the factory. Both of them. Forty years apiece. They'd retired at the same time, five years ago. They'd planned to move to Arizona.

Arizona! Ha! Anna couldn't even go around the block without getting lost. Imagine what would happen if they went to Arizona! She'd probably wind up in the middle of the desert with Sam searching for her. They'd both die of sunstroke.

She'd forgotten how to cook, too. Anna had always been such a good cook. Nothing fancy—just your basic meat and potatoes. But good meat and good potatoes. And always ready when Sam was hungry. They used to love to eat. After work, Anna would cook a big meal, then maybe they'd watch the news on TV, then go over to their daughter's house and spend some time with the grandchildren. They did that, that is, until their daughter's husband got transferred to Germany. That ended that.

Now Sam and Anna didn't eat at home much anymore except when Sam did the cooking, and Sam hated to cook. Never could figure out how to poach an egg just right or even make a good cup of coffee. And he did like his poached eggs and coffee.

Cooking, cleaning, paying the bills. All these things Sam had to do now, if he wanted them done at all. *Too much*, he thought. *Too much.*

"When we gonna get there? When we gonna get there?"

Anna snapped Sam out of his musings as the car turned into the diner driveway, seven miles from home.

"We're here, Hon, we're here."

"Good. Let's eat," said Anna.

Sam opened his door, went around the car, and helped Anna out. She brushed off his hand as if it were a fly and ran up the steps of the diner.

"Hi, Sam. Hi, Anna. Want a menu?" asked Bill, the owner.

"No. You know we don't need one," Sam said as they sat down in the booths by the row of windows.

"Menu. Menu. Menu," said Anna.

"Oh, all right. Give us a menu. She can look. I'll order."

"Looks like she's been putting on some weight again. You too. Guess that's good, huh, Sam?" said Bill.

"Yeah," said Sam. "Anna never eats much when we're home. Guess she doesn't like my cooking. Guess that's why you're still in business, because of people like us."

"So what'll it be today?"

"The usual. Two hot beef sandwiches. A large order of fries. Two coffees. One decaf."

"No," said Anna, peering over her menu and glaring at her husband. "No. No. No."

"Oh, I almost forgot," said Sam. "And two big pieces of chocolate pie."

Anna smiled.

"Give me the menu, Anna," said Sam.

"No. No. No. No."

"That's all right, Sam. She can keep it."

"Thanks, Bill. Give her something to look at while we're waiting. Give her something to read. She always did like to read. I wonder what went wrong? What went wrong?"

Mixed Up

"My mind is all mixed up. Like this," my mother once said to me, holding up a tangled purple strand of yarn she was attempting to crochet into one of her famous afghans.

Mixed up. Tangled. Like a skein of yarn that's slowly being unraveled by a precocious kitten. That's a fairly accurate picture of what happens to someone suffering from Alzheimer's disease.

Alzheimer's is not a normal result of aging. It's related to a specific disease process. Very distinct pathological changes take place in the brain. Under a microscope these changes *do* resemble a tangled skein of yarn.

When someone we love is "all mixed up" because of a confusion-causing disease like Alzheimer's, it's important to have as much information as possible to better understand the disease process. But to understand what goes wrong, we first need to take a look at what's normal. How are our brains supposed to work? How are they structured? Just what *does* go on in our heads, anyway?

The brain is, quite literally, the headquarters for the rest of the body. It's the main office, the control tower, the central meeting place for a vast network of nerves that control all our conscious activity and affect our unconscious actions as well.

The brain isn't much to look at. On the surface it rather resembles a three-pound walnut. But beneath the gray and convoluted exterior of the brain is housed a complex information storage and retrieval system that is responsible for memory, thoughts, language, behavior, and emotions.

The brain consists of three main parts: the cerebrum, or large brain; the cerebellum, or small brain; and the brain stem.

The *cerebrum* fills nearly the entire brain cavity and consists of two cerebral hemispheres covered by a gray outer covering called the *cerebral cortex*. This "gray matter" is associated with our higher mental functions.

The *cerebellum*, located at the back of the brain cavity and below the cerebrum, is responsible for balance and coordinates muscular activity.

The *brain stem* connects the brain to the spinal column and controls the vital functions of breathing and circulation.

To illustrate how a normal brain works, and to better understand what goes wrong when a person becomes afflicted with Alzheimer's, let's look at one specific activity our brains are engaged in every day: making decisions.

The brain, like the rest of our organs, is made up of billions of microscopic cells. In the brain these cells are called *neurons*. Each neuron has a round cell body inside it called a *cell nucleus*. Each cell nucleus sends out short, branching shoots called *dendrites* through one side of its neuron. These free-floating branches are called *dendrite receivers*. The other side of the neuron branches out into *transmitter dendrites* that are gathered together and funneled through a long, threadlike structure called an *axon*.

Let's say we decide to visit a neighbor.

We can't do this with our feet alone. They won't move by themselves. We have to communicate our desire to take a walk to our brain. Our brain passes the message on to our feet.

The message to walk to the neighbor's house is transmitted by an electrical impulse originating in one or more of the cell nuclei. This impulse passes through the transmitter dendrites, through the axon, and on into the terminal shoots or branches that pop out through the end of the axon.

At the end of each cluster of terminal transmitter dendrite branches is a space or gap called a *synapse*.

Once the electrical impulse from our message reaches this synapse, it somehow has to bridge it and communicate with the dendrite receivers of a neighboring neuron. The impulse does this by stimulating the release of chemicals called *neurotransmitters*. There are many different neurotransmitters. One important one is acetylcholine. Acetylcholine is believed to be responsible for, or plays a major role in, thinking and remembering, and is especially important in the processing of recent or short-term memory.[1]

Once the neurotransmitters are released, they pass through the synaptic space and are attached to the surface of the dendrite receivers at specific locations known as *receptors*. This stimulates the release of a high-energy chemical that switches on the electrical impulse in the next neuron along the path.

The brain then tells our feet to take a walk.

This process of message transmission in the brain is indeed beautiful, a lot like a finely crocheted afghan. It is evidence that the brain, like the rest of us, is fearfully and wonderfully made, a complex creation knit together by a loving and imaginative Creator, enabling us to function in amazing ways.

What Goes Wrong?

> I tried to explain it to him so he would understand. I told my husband that having Alzheimer's was like having a car with its wires disconnected. I told him they hadn't figured out a way yet to reconnect the wires in his brain. He seemed to accept that.

> I think my son described it best. He said there's a whole lot of switches in the brain and, one by one, they go.

My husband started acting really weird the summer of 1979. By November he was worse. I tried to get him to go to the doctor but he refused.

He would always shower in the morning. If he was active, he'd shower in midday. He'd also shower at night. But that fall he let himself go and didn't shower at all. He wouldn't even change his clothes. He seemed deeply depressed. If I said anything to him about what he was doing, or not doing, he would get angry. I knew there was something wrong, and he knew there was something wrong, but he wouldn't admit it.

One day our son happened to be visiting. He said, "You know, some of the things you're doing aren't *you*. Don't you think Mother ought to make an appointment for you to see a doctor?"

I guess my husband needed to hear it from our son, because he came back into the house later that day and said, "You're right. I've got to see a doctor. I've got to find out what's wrong with me."

The country was Germany. The year was 1906. He was a psychiatrist and neuropathologist. She was a middle-aged housewife who had experienced profound memory loss, disorientation, confusion, depression, insomnia, and hallucinations. He was her physician. She was his patient.

She died in a mental asylum at age fifty-five. He decided to conduct an autopsy.

When Dr. Alois Alzheimer looked in his microscope and, using a special silver stain, examined a slice of his patient's brain tissue, he discovered two startling abnormalities, inside and outside the brain cells.

Tissue lying inside the cell bodies or nuclei of neurons exhibited an abnormally high number of fine nerve fibers, or filaments, twisted around each other. Dr. Alzheimer called these twisted fibers *neurofibrillary tangles*.

He also saw unusually high numbers of fibrous plaques located between brain cells, composed of degenerating terminal dendrites or burned-out nerve endings that surrounded fibrous waste products of a starchlike amyloid protein. These abnormalities were known as *senile* or *neuritic plaques*. They had been identified before in the autopsied brain tissue of much older people.

For many years after 1906, it was believed that this characteristic tangle and plaque configuration occurred primarily in people under the age of sixty-five; Alzheimer's disease was thought to be a "presenile dementia." Anyone exhibiting signs of confusion after the age of sixty-five was simply labeled "senile," or was said to have a chronic organic brain syndrome, more commonly known as COBS.

This senility of old age was universally blamed on faulty blood circulation or so-called hardening of the arteries, and it was thought to be due to an atherosclerotic process of cholesterol buildup in the arteries of the brain.

But in succeeding years, research finally caught up with reality. In the 1960s, as British researchers began comparing the brains of younger, deceased dementia victims with those of older victims, the electron microscope proved what many had suspected all along: the primary cause of dementia-like symptoms in both younger and older victims was, in fact, one and the same. And it wasn't as rare a phenomenon as previously thought.

Investigators believed the fibrous plaques and neurofibrillary tangles disrupted the passage of neurochemical signals between neurons, resulting in memory loss and impaired thought processes.

In general, the greater the number of plaques, tangles, and associated cellular death, the greater the degree of disturbance in intellectual function. These changes in the brain took place over time and were responsible for the progressive nature of the disease. And while there was a decrease in blood flow to the brain in victims of Alzheimer's disease, this decrease was not caused by atherosclerosis but by brain-cell death brought on by the Alzheimer's process.

In the 1970s, researchers discovered another abnormality associated with Alzheimer's disease, one specifically related to neurochemical changes and the neurotransmitter acetylcholine, normally manufactured in the brain by an enzyme known as *choline acetyltransferase*.

In autopsied brain tissue of people who have the characteristic plaques and tangles, choline acetyltransferase and acetylcholine are missing or present in decreased amounts. Without the stimulus for neurotransmission, signals (messages) are unable to move across the synaptic gap from neuron to neuron. When nerve cells can't communicate with each other, trouble occurs.

This neurochemical loss, as well as the appearance of plaques and tangles, occurs primarily in two areas of the brain: the cortex and the hippocampus.

The cortex, or outer surface of the brain's cerebrum, is composed of those cell bodies that enable us to reason, remember, and speak. In addition to experiencing the neurochemical loss, the cortex of Alzheimer's victims usually shrinks or atrophies, decreasing the brain's surface area.

The hippocampus is a small cluster of cells located in the temporal lobe. It is extremely important to short-term memory function and is also part of the limbic system. This system, activated by motivated behavior and arousal, influences both the hormones and the autonomic motor system, which controls involuntary body functions. It has been called "the seat of our emotions."

What is actually responsible for the development of plaques, tangles, and the death of acetylcholine-producing cells is unknown. Researchers around the world are exploring possible causes or combinations of causes that include genetic factors, a slow virus, abnormalities in the immune system, infectious agents, toxic substances in the environment, metabolic deficits, and abnormalities in DNA repair. Appendix C includes a more detailed overview of research related to causation.

Today Alzheimer's and the senility associated with old age are categorized as one and the same process. They are generally referred to as presenile dementia or senile dementia of the Alzheimer's type, depending on the age of onset. The former usually occurs before age sixty-five; the latter, after.

Our brains are indeed fearfully and wonderfully made, but sometimes things do go wrong with this complex computer that controls us; things we struggle to understand.

Seeing the Symptoms

"Hindsight is always better than foresight," acknowledged one caregiver. "I think the reason I didn't see my wife's symptoms earlier was because I was with her all the time. The changes were so subtle, so gradual."

Probably the most remarkable thing about the very early stages of Alzheimer's disease is its unremarkableness. Signs and symptoms seem to creep up and take us unaware, surprising both us and our loved ones. With the passage of time, the mental and physical deterioration of Alzheimer's becomes more and more pronounced.

While no two people progress at the same rate or according to the same exact pattern, there are some characteristic behavior and personality changes peculiar to each stage of the illness. Knowing what these changes are can help you promote a better quality of life for both yourself and your loved one. Understanding the signs and symptoms of Alzheimer's is a crucial key to caring.[2]

Two to four years is the average length of the first stage of Alzheimer's. The initial symptoms of Alzheimer's may include any or all of the following changes.

Memory loss. Recent events are forgotten. The ability to concentrate, learn new things, and process new information is progressively lost. Bills go unpaid or are paid several times. Checking accounts are overdrawn when the person has trouble adding, subtracting, and balancing a checkbook. The names of known and loved persons may also be forgotten.

People with Alzheimer's usually compensate, initially, by writing notes to themselves. But as the disease progresses, they no longer remember the notes. People frequently deny experiencing these symptoms or rationalize them away as they struggle to preserve their self-esteem and identity.

Confusion and disorientation. Confusion is often related to place and time. People with Alzheimer's sometimes get lost on their way somewhere, or they will arrive at a place and not know where they are or how to get home. The day and month are forgotten as well.

Speech and language disturbances. There may be a progressive inability to name objects or to end sentences. The person searches for words and phrases. Wrong words and phrases are substituted for the forgotten right ones, a condition known as *confabulation. Circumlocution* may also occur, where more words than necessary are used to express an idea.

Impaired judgment. There's a lack of insight and a growing inability to discriminate, understand, and follow directions. Driving is progressively impaired; the person may go through stop signs or wind up going the wrong way on one-way streets. The ability to read is retained but not the ability to understand what is read.

Difficulty completing familiar tasks. It becomes increasingly difficult to cook, clean, engage in familiar hobbies, hold down a job. Routine activities of daily living go through a process of "unlearning." For example, the ability to tie shoes, button a blouse or shirt, or make a cup of coffee may be impaired.

Personality and mood changes. Depression frequently accompanies the early stage of Alzheimer's. There may be listlessness, apathy, suspiciousness, paranoia, social withdrawal, and episodes of crying. Conversely, there may be restlessness, anxiety, agitation, and feelings of "going crazy." On the one hand, people deny the severity of their symptoms, while on the other, they recognize that something's wrong.

Carelessness and neglect. Personal hygiene can become a problem, and people may appear careless or unkempt. They may neglect to bathe, brush their teeth, change, or wash their clothes. They simply may have forgotten how.

Following a diagnosis, caregivers usually ask their loved one's physician, "How long do we have? How many months or years?" There is always a need to know.

The time from the onset of Alzheimer's to the person's death varies greatly. It may be a few years or over twenty, depending on any number of other health-related factors. Generally speaking, the younger a person is, the faster the progression and deterioration.

Facing the Second Stage

"There are some lucid moments, but they are few and far between and they seem to be getting farther and farther away from each other," reported one caregiver whose wife had been diagnosed with Alzheimer's five years earlier.

As Alzheimer's disease progresses, early stage-one symptoms intensify. Memory loss becomes more profound. Behavior becomes more disturbing, bizarre, and unpredictable. This second stage of Alzheimer's may last for two to ten years.

We need to keep in mind that not all victims of Alzheimer's will experience the same symptoms, but there are some behavior changes common to dementia.

Continued and progressive memory loss. Past events as well as recent ones may no longer be remembered. The ability to engage in familiar hobbies or carry out even the routine activities of daily living, such as bathing, dressing, and toileting, is impaired.

Progressive to complete disorientation and confusion. Our loved ones may lose their ability to recognize people, including family members. They may not recognize their own reflection in a mirror. They may forget the names and uses of familiar objects. They may wander off and get lost, or they may even get lost in their own homes.

Speech, communication, and language disorders. People with second-stage Alzheimer's are progressively unable to express themselves and to complete sentences. The repetition of words, questions, and phrases is common. Speech may become garbled or very slow.

Catastrophic reactions. These may include pronounced mood swings or personality changes, including outbursts of anger, increased suspiciousness or paranoia, and even episodes of physical violence, usually short-lived.

Wandering, restlessness, and pacing. Restless wandering often occurs at night or in the late afternoon, around sundown. Repetitious movements, such as finger or foot tapping, lip smacking, and constant chewing motions, may increase.

Various behavior problems. There may be hallucinations or delusions of being persecuted. People with Alzheimer's frequently hide and hoard things and may tear the house apart looking for "lost" items. There may be inappropriate sexual and social behavior with marked social withdrawal.

Physical signs. Motor activity may be affected; many people in the second stage progressively lose their ability to engage in activities requiring hand and finger coordination. Opening a can with a can opener, buttoning a shirt, tying a shoelace, hammering a nail—all could be affected. Occasionally there is muscle twitching or jerking. People may tend to lose their balance and fall as coordination becomes impaired. Eating and elimination problems manifest themselves.

The following chapters highlight some of the more common and difficult management problems caregivers have identified, along with suggestions for dealing with these problems in the varying stages of the disease. Late-stage symptoms include an intensification of stage-two symptoms that gradually progress into a need for total care. The last chapter of this book discusses care needs of people in the final stage of Alzheimer's.

Part Two

CARING FOR YOUR LOVED ONE

We can do no great things—
only small things with great love.

Mother Teresa

Chapter 5

When Memory Starts to Fade

"The gifts of God for the people of God. Take them in remembrance that Christ died for you, and feed on him in your hearts by faith, with thanksgiving."

Father Joe walked slowly down the row of communicants, pausing before each of his parishioners to say the familiar words. "The body of Christ, the bread of heaven. The body of Christ, the bread of heaven. The body of Christ, the bread of heaven."

When he came to the last kneeling person, he paused and smiled. Here was Mary again, just as she had been for the past eight months.

Mary. A seventy-five-year-old woman who had never married, and a charter member of the church. A Sunday school teacher for forty years until she was sixty-five, at which time she told everyone she was tired, retired, and ready to relax. "You folks take over," said Mary. "I'll sit and enjoy church."

Mary, whose habits the past eight months had become rather unusual. She had developed a weekly pattern of bringing her luggage—two overstuffed suitcases held together with string and adhesive tape—to church. She'd even carry them up to the altar and set them down, one on each side of her. Father Joe once asked Mary where she was going with her suitcases. Mary glared at him and told him it was none of his business.

Today, Mary wasn't exactly dressed for church, not for church on a warm summer morning, at any rate. She had on her bulky gray overcoat with the unraveling hem and what appeared to be several layers of thick wool stockings. A pair of fur-lined boots graced her feet. One toe stuck out through a hole.

It wasn't as if Mary had to wear these clothes, thought Father Joe. The ladies of the church had offered to take her shopping. They'd even purchased some new summer clothes for her and had delivered them in person. But Mary wouldn't let them in the house, telling them she didn't accept charity and to please give the clothes to the poor. "I'm fine," Mary insisted. "Fine."

And Mary was fine, to a point. The senior nutrition program delivered two meals a day to her—one hot, one cold—so she was at least eating a balanced diet. But Mary never let the volunteers in the house, insisting they leave the food wrapped in a brown paper bag on the porch. By every morning the previous day's meals had disappeared, and the dirty dishes were back in the paper bag on the porch.

The county nurses were aware of Mary's situation and were also trying to help. They sent an aide to clean her house, but Mary wouldn't let the aide inside. She insisted, through the keyhole, that she was fine. "My house is clean," she told the aide.

"It sure didn't smell fine and clean through the keyhole!" the aide told her supervisor. "But what could I do?"

Today, though, Mary's clothes and Mary's house really didn't matter. Mary was here in church, and she was ready to receive communion.

As Father Joe bent down to place the wafer in Mary's mouth, he thought he could detect the faint odor of urine floating up and mingling its ammonia with the aroma of burning incense.

But Mary wasn't aware of this. Her eyes were closed in an attitude of prayer. Her mouth was open to receive the wafer. And her hands gripped the handles of her two packed suitcases.

Of all of us gathered here today, thought Father Joe, *Mary is probably the most prepared to enter the heavenly kingdom.*

The Faces of Memory Loss

Several weeks before I completed the final draft of the first edition of this book, the father of a member of our support group died. I went to the viewing at the funeral parlor, where my friend and I stood next to her father's casket, talking about the final, emotionally charged days of his life.

As I was about to leave, my friend turned to me and said, "Be sure to tell people that Alzheimer's is more than a little memory loss. It's not just forgetting names or how to balance your checkbook. It's forgetting everything, eventually. Everything you ever did that was important to who you were as a person. Everyone you've ever known. Write about that. People need to know."

My friend was right. People do need to know. For with knowledge comes understanding and the ability to empathize with caregivers faced with a responsibility that may last anywhere from one to over twenty years. As caregivers ourselves, we need knowledge and understanding to be able to deal with the many faces of Alzheimer's, especially the many faces of memory loss.

My own mother was an artist. Not a professional artist, but an artist nonetheless. My most vivid childhood memories are of Mom sitting in her living room rocker each evening after supper, in front of an old easel my father had made, surrounded by little tubes of oil paint or boxes of pastels. Mom was always in the middle of a painting project.

Later in life my mother packed up her paints and pastels and switched to crocheting. With her artist's eye she wove thousands of granny squares into dozens of beautiful afghans. When she first started having symptoms of Alzheimer's, she continued to crochet. In fact, her afghans were one of the first signs that anything was wrong.

I came home for a visit one Christmas and Mom had one of her latest creations spread out on the bed. It basically looked okay, much the same as all her other variegated blue and white afghans. This one, however, also contained a few isolated squares of green and white. When I mentioned it, my mother just shrugged. "Looks okay to me," I remember her saying. That did not show an artist's appraising eye, and it was not her usual attitude. My mother always liked her afghans to be perfect, and she would tear them apart and start them over if they weren't.

As the months passed, Mom continued to crochet, but the granny squares gradually became circles, then chains and, finally, bunches of tangled yarn. Unlike many people with Alzheimer's who become frustrated with the loss of their ability to continue to engage in well loved hobbies, Mom seemed content to do what she could and was generally oblivious to the fact that her abilities were deteriorating.

My husband forgot how to dress himself. He couldn't figure out how to button his shirt, tie his shoes, or buckle his belt. He just couldn't seem to figure out what went where.

Dad had a colostomy and had always done his own irrigating, but it got to the point where he couldn't remember how to do it. So my mother started to do it for him. Then, eventually, the public health nurse came in because Dad wouldn't let my mother touch him.

The hardest part each morning was trying to brush Mom's teeth. She simply couldn't figure out what to do with the toothbrush. I'd put some toothpaste on the brush and try to show her what I wanted her to do but after a while it was useless. I had to brush them for her if I wanted them brushed at all.

One of the most difficult and painful behavior changes caregivers have to face is the loss of their loved ones' memory of self as they fail to recognize themselves.

One morning my mother was sitting in her rocking chair in the bedroom while I cleaned out a closet in the hall. All of a sudden I heard her crying and rushed into the bedroom to see what was the matter. She was looking in the mirror repeating the same phrase over and over again: "I lost myself. I lost myself."

No less painful is the realization that our loved ones don't seem to know us and may have delusions that we are someone else.

I remember one day my mother said to my dad, "She wants me to sit down. Who is she? Do you know who she is?"

If there was anything left of my heart to break, it broke right there. I walked into our back yard and cried my eyes out.

It got to the point that my father didn't recognize my mother. He thought she was a stranger and would lock her out of the house.

If their dog needed to go out at night, my mother had to go out the kitchen door and onto the porch to let the dog out the porch door. Sometimes Dad would get up and lock the kitchen door behind her, and then he wouldn't let her back in. Twenty-four hours a day she had to wear a skeleton key around her neck.

My wife finally decided I didn't belong to her. I wasn't her husband. I had no business being in the bedroom with her.

She would rant and rave and carry on about the strange man in her room and kept telling me she didn't have to sleep in the same room with a man.

I told her I wouldn't touch her, that I was just there if she needed help, but she said she didn't need me and was perfectly able to take care of herself.

I used to have to wait until she was asleep to go to bed myself. Do you know how that made me feel?

Some people with Alzheimer's retain some recognition of themselves far into the disease but have no idea who others are or where they are. Many continue to live in memories of the past.

Anna Wilcox resided on the skilled unit of a nursing home where I worked. She was always certain of her identity, if not the time or the place. If you asked her name, she'd declare with authority and in a very loud voice, "My name is Anna Wilcox!" But if you asked her if she knew where she was, she'd usually say she was in Ohio, teaching a class of fifteen students in a one-room schoolhouse. The year was somewhere around 1939.

In the evenings after I'd given her medication and turned out her light, she'd tell me about the school. I didn't try to reorient her to reality. At Anna's stage of dementia, reality orientation usually doesn't work. It only frustrates. So instead, I asked her to tell me about the school in Ohio and the children she taught. And she did.

Often it didn't make much sense. She rambled a lot and sometimes mixed up her role as a schoolteacher with her role as a waitress, another job she apparently held for a time. But it really didn't matter at nine o'clock at night. I'd rub her back a little, listen to her stories. Soon she'd be fast asleep with a smile on her face, dreaming, I like to think, about the past.

Simple Memory Joggers

There are many faces of memory loss with Alzheimer's disease. As caregivers we need to accept and acknowledge them, then help our loved ones deal with them one by one, a day at a time, as the disease progresses.

Here are a few suggestions. Some of these initial ideas can be utilized with the loved one who is still living at home in the early stages of the disease. Others can be helpful as the disease progresses and the ability to read and comprehend written instructions is lost.

➤ A large wall calendar can help a person keep track of time. Hang a marker nearby so the days can be crossed off as they pass.

➤ Provide a simple list of the day's activities in the order in which they should occur. For example, 1. Eat breakfast. 2. Take green pill with milk. 3. Feed cat.

➤ Post the list in a conspicuous place. Some people with early dementia prefer note cards with memory-jogging information on them about tasks to complete, phone numbers to remember, and so on. These can be kept in a small file box with dividers for different subjects.

➤ If telling time is a problem, consider switching to digital clocks. It's easier to read the time than to figure it out. This technique completely cured my mother of asking "What time is it?" literally dozens of times a day, and it greatly relieved her stress and anxiety. We put digital clocks in the bedroom, living room, and kitchen.

➤ Pill boxes labeled for the day of the week and time of day are available in pharmacies and home-care supply stores. These can be effective in the early stages of Alzheimer's if your loved one, though still able personally to take medication, might mix up pill bottles. Some people create their own pill boxes with egg cartons. You or a community-health nurse will need to refill and monitor this system on a regular basis.

➤ Avoid moving things around in the house. Having things in familiar places is an aid to memory, as is keeping to a familiar routine.

➤ Pictures and/or labels may help a person identify various rooms in the house. For example, if your loved one has trouble finding the bathroom, color code the door or put a sign on it identifying it as the bathroom. As the disease progresses you may need to switch to a picture of a tub or toilet.

➤ Some nursing homes have the names or photographs of confused residents outside their rooms. You might also do this in the home. If your loved one can no longer recognize a personal photograph, hang some type of identifying article of clothing such as an old familiar hat or sweater. My mom began to identify her bedroom when we hung a picture of her grandmother and grandfather next to the door. Prior to that, she kept getting lost.

➤ Labels on various items in the home—hot and cold water faucets and the contents of drawers—can also help jog the memory. Again, as the disease progresses, you might switch from large written labels to pictures of actual drawer contents.

➤ Let habit be your helper. Your loved one may still be able to perform many routine tasks of daily living with a little help from you. Often the problem lies in initiating the activity. Once it is started, habit seems to take over, and routine tasks can continue to be carried out.

For example, you may have to put the toothpaste on the brush, hold the brush to your loved one's mouth and begin brushing. He or she then may be able to finish the job. Or you may have to cut up food, place some food on a fork and guide hand to mouth a couple of times until the connection is made. Maintain independence for as long as possible for both your sakes.

Maintaining People Awareness

Spend time with your loved one reminiscing. Reminiscence, or life review, is a technique frequently used in adult homes and nursing homes for older people without dementia. It may also be a helpful intervention for people in the early stages of dementia.

Talking about people and events from the past, flipping through old photo albums, reading aloud old letters from friends and relatives, looking at old mementos—all of these activities can help maintain some awareness of self and others. They can also serve to draw you and your loved one closer together. Old familiar songs or hymns that have been an important part of your loved one's life can be used in all stages of the disease. This "music therapy" can be particularly valuable in the later stages, especially at night.

Trying to convince people with Alzheimer's that you aren't who they think you are, or that you are who they think you aren't, is probably futile. It may simply provoke a catastrophic or emotional reaction. During nonstressful times, however (and there will be many), remind your loved one of who you are. Say his or her name frequently, too. Our names are important. They're part of our identity. For Alzheimer's sufferers, they can quickly be lost.

Your loved one may revert, at various times, to living in the past. As the disease progresses, trying to reorient to reality may no longer work. A better approach may often be to help your loved one focus attention on events from the past and the feelings associated with them.

We all live in the past to a certain extent. We all spend some time daily remembering various events, both good and bad, that were important to us. These events evoke memories and feelings that make us glad or sad. We might assume that the same happens to our loved ones. Instead of getting upset and trying to orient them to the present, we need to help them focus on these events. They may need to talk about them and express their feelings.[1]

Thingamajigs and Thingamabobs

Two of my mother's favorite words when I was growing up were *thingamajig* and *thingamabob*. You could always use those words in a pinch if you couldn't remember the name of something. They were handy words. We liked them.

As Mom's disease progressed, virtually everything became a "thingamajig" or "thingamabob." It became increasingly difficult for her to name familiar objects, to complete sentences, and, finally, to communicate any thoughts whatsoever.

Language loss as well as memory loss is common in Alzheimer's disease. One frequent behavior pattern is the substitution of wrong words for right words, especially at the end of a sentence.

> One of the first symptoms we noticed early in the progression of my wife's disease was word substitution. This continued for a long time. She'd say something like "I need to go out and get the bird" when she meant she had to go out and get the mail. Or she needed to "cook the car" when she meant she needed to cook dinner. I could usually figure out what she meant, but she sure confused a lot of other people.

Some people can manage to express a few words of a sentence but not the complete thought. Their communication may sound as if they are reading out of an old first-grade primer where all the words are nouns and verbs.

> My husband's conversation became short and clipped. He'd say "go" when he wanted to go for a ride, "eat" when he was hungry, and "love" when he wanted to hug or be hugged.

The ability to complete sentences may be lost.

> My wife would start a sentence. She'd get three or four words out, and the rest was just gibberish. It used to make me feel so bad because I didn't know what she was trying to tell me. She looked so earnest. I would say, "Is that right?" And that seemed to please her even though it didn't satisfy me.

> Once in a while a word comes out I can understand, like "Christmas," or a phrase like "It's cold in here." But most of the time my husband just babbles. Sometimes we sit and babble together. I love to hear his voice. I dread the day when his babbling stops. Can you understand that?

Repetitive or perseverative speech is a frequent problem and, for caregivers, can be one of the most annoying symptoms of the disease. Words, phrases, and questions are often repeated over and over again.

> My wife kept repeating herself until I thought I'd go crazy. Sometimes it was the same word. But the worst thing was the same question—"What time is it? What time is it? What time is it?" And I always felt I had to answer her.

Sometimes people with dementia revert to the language of their youth, or language may fail altogether.

> In the nursing home my father reverted to his childhood language. His mother came from Czechoslovakia and they always

talked the Bohemian language at home. For one period of time, when he was still able to talk, he kept bouncing back and forth between English and Bohemian. It drove the aides crazy.

Now my father can't even form words to talk to me. It's like his tongue is three times its normal size. He tries to say something once in a while but no intelligible word will come out.

If I say, "Dad, are you okay?" he may shake his head yes or no. Then again, he may not.

Breaking through the Walls

Language losses are not easy to deal with, but the following tips may help facilitate both giving and receiving information as you learn new ways to communicate.

➤ Face your loved one when speaking and maintain eye contact. Speak slowly and distinctly and lower the pitch of your voice. This is especially important if there is any hearing impairment. A low voice is more important than a loud voice.

➤ Ask questions or give directions one at a time. Don't expect immediate responses. Give your loved one time to process the information before answering or actively responding. If your loved one is trying to respond verbally but is becoming frustrated, help out. You may need to finish a sentence or supply a word. Help to decrease anxiety.

➤ Tune in to your loved one's body language. Listen to what is being said by facial expressions, body movements, posture, and so forth.

If your loved one is trying to communicate something but can't verbally express it, try asking simple questions that can be answered with yes, no, or a head movement. If you suspect your loved one is in pain, you may have to point to or touch the area you think might be hurting. Ask for a response with a nod of the head, to see if you are correct.

➤ Look for possible contributing causes for repetitious verbalizations or behaviors. For example, "oh, oh, oh" repeated over and over may be because of pain or the need to go to the bathroom. Sometimes you can determine no underlying reason for the behavior, even though your loved one seems anxious and troubled. If you say "It's okay" or "It's all right" and show affection, you may help the sufferer feel less anxious and more secure.

Though there are no sure cures, music may also be helpful for curbing repetition. Sarah White, a nursing-home resident diagnosed with Alzheimer's, constantly tapped her foot on the floor and her fingers on the arm of her wheelchair. She also repeated, "I'm lost, I'm lost, I'm lost."

One day we discovered that Sarah had been a minister's wife and a minister's daughter. Church attendance had been a regular part of her life, but no one knew it at the home. So we began taking her to weekly church services. As soon as she heard the music playing and the congregation singing, Sarah stopped her repetitious tapping, except to keep time to the music. She also stopped saying, "I'm lost."

We finally got a radio for Sarah's room and kept it tuned to a religious or a classical music station. The music seemed to soothe her, and the repetitious, perseverative behavior and verbalizations diminished.

If all your attempts to intervene and break the cycle of repetition fail, you may have to simply remove yourself from the scene for a while to keep from blowing your cool. Pray for patience to weather it until next time.

The many faces of memory loss are indeed painful to see, but the losses can be lessened as we look for ways to preserve and enhance the memory that still exists.

Chapter 6

Emotional Fireworks

One dictionary definition of *catastrophe* is "a sudden, violent change, such as an earthquake." This well describes the various catastrophic reactions that frequently accompany Alzheimer's, ranging from the slight tremor of anxiety to a sometimes violent verbal or physical outburst.

> We never fought when I was growing up. My mother was very sweet, gentle, and easygoing. But we fought when she got Alzheimer's.

Catastrophic reactions are hard to understand. A closer look, however, can often indicate some underlying reasons for our loved one's bizarre behavior. We need to be aware of the various pressure points that might suddenly trigger an emotional eruption.

Triggers for Catastrophic Reactions

Catastrophic reactions can occur when our loved one is frustrated by diminishing abilities.

> My dad had been an excellent mechanic. But it got to the point where he ruined everything he touched. It was the most pitiful thing to see.
>
> I'll never forget one experience. Dad's Jeep was sitting in the garage and he was tinkering with it, trying to get it to run. He finally came running into the house, absolutely beside himself.

"I can't do it," he was crying. "I can't do it. Would you fix my Jeep? Would you fix my Jeep?" That broke my heart.

Reactions can sometimes be triggered by irrational fears. They may be accompanied by paranoia.

The community-health nurse would try to give my husband a bath or even just wash him, and he'd fight. You couldn't struggle with him because you'd lose. He had the strength of a bull. He wouldn't let anyone near him. He'd say that the water was cold, that he was afraid of it.

My mother was absolutely terrified one evening, and she kept pointing to the double door on our deck. I was sure someone was out there, but then I realized she was seeing her own reflection in the glass. I remembered to keep the drapes closed after that episode.

Once, when my mother was still driving, she looked in the rear-view mirror and really got hysterical. She was sure the person in the car behind us was following us.

The person in the car was my brother!

Catastrophic reactions can sometimes be triggered by specific actions on the part of another person, especially if the other person is perceived as a threat in any way.

If my father felt threatened he would pinch or hit, especially if you tried to get him to do something he didn't want to.

One night I had to take my mother to the hospital for a medical emergency, and a friend of mine stayed with my father.

My father kept wanting to go to the hospital too, and he tried to get in the car. He hit my friend over the head with a flashlight three times when she tried to stop him.

Reactions can occur when we try to get our loved one to choose among various options or respond to several questions at once.

I remember taking my father to restaurants. I was trying to make him feel better about himself, so I would always ask him to choose what he wanted to eat; I wanted to give him a choice. But instead of feeling better he became frustrated and upset because there were too many things to choose from. He couldn't process all that information, and once he even started to cry. When I finally understood what was happening, we still went out, but I simply ordered for us both.

Catastrophic reactions usually seem like marked personality changes. They are sometimes accompanied by outpourings of profanity and verbal abuse, directed at us. Occasionally they turn into physical violence.

My husband got mean, real mean, and he was never mean in his life. He even punched me once with his fists.

One minute my wife seems to know who we are, and five minutes later she'll be yelling and calling us names. It's just as if somebody turns a switch and another person appears. She gets violent and very abusive, just the opposite of what she used to be. She was one of the most lovable people. There wasn't enough she could do for other people. Not enough. And she never swore. But since she's developed Alzheimer's, I've learned language from her I didn't know existed.

It's a natural tendency to respond to our loved one's catastrophic reactions with emotional outbursts of our own. Catastrophic reactions are stressful and emotionally charged experiences, and if we're feeling unduly stressed to begin with, we will react rather than respond. But if we do that, we're in for trouble. As soon as the episode is over, we'll feel like a failure because of the way we handled the situation.

The key phrase to remember when confronted with a catastrophic reaction on the part of a loved one is *keep cool.* That may seem difficult if not impossible to do given the circumstances, but it is the best advice we can give ourselves. It will help to divert disaster and convert catastrophes into experiences we and our loved ones will be able to live through.

What to Do and What to Avoid

The following dos and don'ts offer some practical suggestions.

Do avoid situations or events which might trigger catastrophic reactions. If you can't avoid them, anticipate them. For example, if you take your loved one grocery shopping, avoid Saturday mornings and Friday nights. Go at times when the store is less likely to be a beehive of people. If you go out to eat, avoid the prime-time hours when restaurants are crowded.

Do make life as predictable as possible. Most of us get tired of the same old grind, but people with dementia find a daily routine secure and comfortable. Marked schedule changes may precipitate catastrophic reactions. Plan your loved one's life as much as possible. This may become less of a problem as the disease progresses.

Do limit choices. Remember that your loved one's ability to discriminate is markedly affected by Alzheimer's. If you are helping your mother or wife dress, for example, asking her to choose the blue, brown, yellow, or white dress may overwhelm her. You might show her two dresses and ask her to choose one. Or you may simply have to choose one for her.

Use simple sentences. Offer one thought at a time. Let one task be completed before talking about another one.

Do simplify the activities of daily living. In the area of clothing, consider substituting pullover dresses, shirts, and sweaters for those that button; slip-on loafers for shoes with laces; and Velcro fasteners for zippers, buttons, and snaps. Such replacements will help your loved one maintain independence for as long as possible while minimizing catastrophic reactions.

Don't talk about your loved one's behavior problems to others in the presence of your loved one. Just because someone may no longer be able to communicate verbally does not mean he or she no longer understands what's going on or what's being said. Think about how you'd feel in a similar situation and be sensitive. Always assume more understanding and comprehension than you actually see.

Don't take personally the things your loved one says. You or other family members may be accused of stealing money, selling the family home, or withdrawing your love. Attempting to deny the accusations may only make things worse.

If accused of stealing money, for example, you might offer to help your loved one search for it. One caregiver I interviewed has a locked box for which she keeps the key. Inside the box are her mother's checkbook, recent bank receipts, and a little cash. If her mother accuses her of theft, they search for the box together. When they "find" it, her mother leafs through the bank stubs and the checkbook and usually concludes that all is intact. The catastrophic reaction blows over.

Don't argue or try to reason. Remember that the disease affects the memory and the mind's ability to think logically. Spouses may not understand why it isn't safe for them to drive the family car. To believe that they will understand if someone just explains it enough times is an error in judgment. Arguments can also make your loved one more suspicious and defensive, attitude changes you don't need.

Instead of arguing and reasoning, *acknowledge and validate*. The disorientation and confusion that are part of Alzheimer's result in more than just bizarre behaviors. Dementia also stirs up deep feelings—for us *and* our loved ones. These feelings seem to have little to do with intellectual impairment. Beneath a belligerent exterior, our loved ones may be nursing a lot of fear, disappointment, and hurt, just as we would if we were frustrated in our attempts to do something we'd always loved to do, something that was an important part of our identity. Helping our loved ones to verbalize those feelings, or even to cry, may be the best thing we can do.

Do avoid shouting or raising your voice. Don't correct or confront the bizarre behavior. A loud, accusatory voice implies that we somehow expect change in the behavior. We need to remember that the behavior is not deliberate. Alzheimer's sufferers don't want to act the way they do.

Avoid the "why" questions: "Why are you doing this" or "Why did you do it?" "Why" questions can put others on the defensive. They feel they have to justify their behavior, which in this case they are not responsible for. The normal reaction to a perceived threat is fight or flight. Both are catastrophic reactions. What our loved ones need most is our love and acceptance of who they are, just the way they are.

Speak softly, treating your loved one with the same dignity and respect you would want to be shown if you were in the same shoes. The Bible says, "A gentle answer quiets anger, but a harsh one stirs it up." (Proverbs 15:1, TEV). Soothing answers and soft tones can temper many a catastrophic reaction.

Do move beyond the event and forget it as quickly as possible. Defuse situations by using a technique called distraction. Distraction might include changing the subject, going for a walk to "search" for the missing item, or offering a favorite food to eat.

Be thankful for your loved one's short-term memory and consider it a blessing in the case of catastrophic reactions.

Don't physically restrain your loved one unless it's absolutely necessary. He or she may feel fenced in and become even more combative.

Instead, capitalize on the excess energy at this time. If your loved one is turning over the living room furniture, it might be an ideal time to clean the rug! Try to redirect the energy and get him or her to help you.

Do consider the possibility that medication, such as a mild tranquilizer, may help your loved one. Catastrophic reactions are often like dormant volcanoes—they suddenly erupt without much warning and are over as quickly as they started. But in some cases the catastrophe may seem continuous. If this is the case for you, talk with your physician about possible medication.

Do remove yourself from emotionally charged situations. If you feel you are going to explode, you probably will. It's no sin to walk away from your loved one if you think the situation is going to get the best of you, or if you anticipate physical violence. If you can do so without endangering anyone's safety, leave the scene for a time and return when everyone has calmed down.

Avoid emotionally distancing yourself. Reach out with a warm embrace, a kiss, a touch of your hand. Affection often can defuse a difficult situation. Touch can communicate that you care. It can offer reassurance and affirmation as well as affection.

"Perfect love drives out all fear" (1 John 4:18, TEV). Our love for our loved ones may not be perfect. In fact, we may feel very unloving at times. But it will ultimately be our love that will drive out the fears we have—and the fears our loved ones have—in dealing with the various catastrophic reactions of Alzheimer's.

Relying on a Greater Power

Sometimes we need to draw on someone other than ourselves, stronger than ourselves, to meet our loved one's needs. This is particularly true in relation to catastrophic reactions.

Several years ago I was working in home care when I got a call in the middle of the night from Mrs. Blake, one of our clients. Her husband, who had Alzheimer's, was having a catastrophic reaction. All six feet and four inches of him was trying desperately to get out of the house. The only thing standing in his way was his four-foot, ten-inch wife. "What do I do?" she asked. "Can you come over?"

My first inclination was to go help, but I knew that would mean delay. At the time my own mother had a tendency to wander at night. I couldn't leave her alone. Getting her up and dressed to go with me would be a major, time-consuming project.

My second inclination was to call the ambulance or the local police. Surely they'd have the manpower to help this poor woman. But when I mentioned it, she said no, she'd rather not have them there. She wanted to handle it alone.

At that point I was stumped. I told her I'd call her back in a few minutes and I hung up the phone, thinking through various strategies.

Then I did something I'd done many times before in similar situations with my own mother. I prayed. I asked God to give Mrs. Blake wisdom and courage, to protect her and her husband from physical harm, and to defuse that explosive situation.

Five minutes later, I called back.

"Goodness!" Mrs. Blake said. "A few minutes after you called, my husband stopped storming around, went over to his chair, and sat down. Now he's sleeping like a baby. I guess we'll be okay."

I guess we will be okay. Talking to God may not be the first thing that comes to our mind in the middle of a catastrophic reaction, but it should definitely be high on our list of therapeutic interventions. We care very much for our loved ones. Prayer can remind us that someone else cares too.

Chapter 7

Always on the Move

I once worked in a nursing home that had a locked ward. All the residents there had some form of dementia, and all were free to roam and wander around. If the wing had not been locked, many simply would have wandered off, including Sam Smith.

Sam was a man in his eighties. In his younger years he had worked as a conductor on the local railroad; when Sam stood by the locked door of the ward, he still looked the part. He wore his old battered conductor's cap and carried a paper sack filled with crackers. "My lunch," he'd say, if anyone asked. And if anyone questioned why he was waiting by the door the same time every day, Sam would smile and say, "Waiting for the train."

When the evening nurses pressed the buzzer on the outside of the door to signal to the day staff they had arrived, Sam would get excited. He thought it was the train whistle.

"Not today, Sam. Not today," the nurses would say as they filed through the door. Sam would continue to pace back and forth by the door. Tomorrow maybe, but not today. Sam would continue to pace back and forth by the door for an hour after the shift change. Then he'd go back to his room and wait for tomorrow's train.

Sundowning

When the sun goes down, people with Alzheimer's frequently want to get up and go. Confusion heightens at this time of day. Restless wandering and agitation increase. The name for this phenomenon is *sundowning*. Sundowning is a common occurrence in nursing homes.

It also occurs at home, and it is often accompanied by catastrophic reactions.

> My wife's restlessness and agitation seem to be worse in the winter months, when the days get shorter and it gets dark early in the afternoon.
>
> Sometimes she gets angry along with getting restless and agitated. Her anger might last half an hour or four or five hours. That big crack in the window over there happened late one afternoon when my wife got angry and threw her shoe.

Reasons for sundowning are unclear, though late afternoon fatigue may be a contributing factor. It's also wise to consider obvious and correctable physical catalysts for odd behavior: hunger, thirst, or the need to go to the bathroom.

If rest, food, drink, or elimination fail to calm your loved one's agitation, here are some things you can do to cope with it.

Simplify the environment. In nursing homes, sundowning frequently occurs during shift changes, when nurses and assistants are coming and going and causing confusion. Some times of day are more confusing than others in the home as well. For example, a younger Alzheimer's victim with school-age children may find after-school time particularly stressful. The kids come home with their friends, the television blares, the house is in an uproar.

You may not be able to change the environment, but you can move your loved one to a room away from busy people traffic. Total isolation isn't always necessary, but quieter surroundings may help decrease stress.

If you're able to provide a "locked ward" type of environment, either in a room of your home or in a fenced area outside, do so. This will enable your loved one to roam at will and, hopefully, work off some excess energy.

Find simple things for your loved one to do. One helpful idea of a "rummage box" comes from a caregiver.

I made up what I call Mary's rummage box. Every afternoon Mary would enter other people's rooms in our adult home and go through their dresser drawers. Needless to say, she wasn't very popular with some of the more alert people.

I got Mary a big box and filled it with soft things like washcloths, towels, balls of yarn, and stuffed animals. Then I sat Mary down at the kitchen table while I got dinner ready. For an hour or so she seemed content just taking the things out of the box one by one and putting them back in. She'd also fold and unfold the towels and washcloths.

Spend time with your loved one. Let him or her be near you. Lack of security may contribute to sundowning. Your loved one may need the reassurance that you, unlike the setting sun, won't leave.

Find easy things to do together that are meaningful and productive: washing and drying dishes, sweeping the floor, folding laundry, cooking dinner. Even if you have to rewash, resweep, refold, or repeel, the fact that you're able to continue sharing in these daily activities is worth the extra time.

Your loved one may not be able to clean the whole house or cook an entire meal, but the loss of these abilities is usually gradual. You can capitalize on the abilities that are still intact and help preserve them for as long as possible. When you do that, you also help preserve your loved one's self-esteem.

If your loved one is manageable, perhaps late afternoon is the best time to grocery shop, do errands, or simply get away from it all. Go for a drive and enjoy the scenery together.

Reliving pleasures from the past may also be a means of calming down a person with Alzheimer's. Consider watching an old movie on television, looking through photo albums, and talking about old times, old friends. Sing some favorite songs or hymns. Put on a record and dance. Do what you used to do. Focus on the familiar.

Late afternoon may also be a good time to take a walk with your loved one. It's good exercise for you both, and you might find that a late afternoon exercise break will decrease nightly wandering and enhance your loved one's ability to sleep.

Sundowning can indeed cause frustration and anxiety for everyone in the family touched by Alzheimer's disease. But it can also be an incentive for new dimensions of creativity and companionship.

Prone to Wander

You'd think a lot of restless wandering throughout the day would exhaust your loved one as much as it does you, but this is not always the case. Many people with Alzheimer's continue to wander well into the night and on into the early hours of the morning.

> I was always on the alert. My husband would get up around 2:00 A.M and turn on the light in our room. He'd pack a suitcase, or sometimes just a box of trinkets, and head downstairs. Sometimes he'd just roll his bedding up and take it downstairs and pile it on the floor. Usually he got dressed.
>
> So then I'd get out of my bed and put my housecoat on and go downstairs with him, and we'd just sit in the living room chairs in the dark until 4:00 or 5:00 A.M. and then we'd both go back to bed for a while. He never tried to go out at night, but he was up for most of it.

> My wife started living in the past, living on the farm where she grew up. She was always getting out of bed in the middle of the night. Then she'd wander all through the house, looking for the animals.

> My husband wandered all over the house at night. I stayed awake to make sure he was all right. The doctor wanted me to tie my husband in bed so I could get some rest, but I just couldn't. And the medications he gave him only seemed to make him worse, especially during the day.

So he wandered and I didn't get much sleep. I finally hired people to stay at night, but that first year was terrible.

If wandering around the house at night is part of your loved one's lifestyle, the following suggestions may be helpful. As always with behavior management problems, think about physical causes first.

➤ Hunger or thirst can contribute to restless wandering. Your loved one may be looking for the refrigerator. Offer a small glass of *warm milk or herbal tea* just before retiring. Avoid anything with caffeine, including hot chocolate. Consider the addition of complex carbohydrate foods, such as a sandwich or crackers and cheese.

➤ On the other hand, what you perceive as restlessness may be the sign of a full bladder. Be sure there is *a trip to the bathroom* before retiring, and watch out for excessive fluid intake for several hours prior to going to bed. You might also try placing a commode in a strategic spot, either at the foot of the bed or in front of the bedroom door if finding the bathroom in the middle of the night presents a problem.

➤ If your loved one suffers from some other malady in addition to Alzheimer's that may cause pain, consider *appropriate pain medication* at night. Pain can contribute to agitation.

➤ Nightly wandering may be a symptom of daily inertia. What may be needed during daylight hours is some sort of *sustained activity,* such as a planned walk or two around the block.[1]

➤ Think about the effect *environmental cues* might have on confused people. If your loved one gets up at night and spies his coat and hat on the chair and his clothes all neatly laid out for the next morning, he may assume it already is the next morning, get up, and get dressed. You also might want to disguise obvious exits with not-so-obvious drapes.

➤ *A warm bath or shower* prior to retiring may help your loved one relax. Avoid bubble baths. They can contribute to urinary tract infections, a complication you don't need. Follow the bath with a soothing back rub.

➤ Keep *a bedside radio* tuned softly to a classical music station or the type of music your loved one has always enjoyed. Some caregivers leave the television turned on low. Experiment if necessary. A talk show may be the perfect soporific.

➤ *Reading* to your loved one from a familiar source may help induce sleep. Many people have been used to reading a book before retiring.

➤ Many nursing homes encourage families to bring in *stuffed animals*. Cuddly things can be comforting and seem to lend a sense of security. This can also work in the home for some people.

➤ *Sleep medication* may be the answer for some, but it should generally be used as a last resort. You will need a prescription for most medications. You might ask your physician for a dosage range and be sure the medication is in a low enough dose to allow you to experiment. Never use more when less will do. If tranquilizers are taken during the day, you might be able to divide them up so the stronger dose can be given at night.

Remember that all medications, including sleep medications, have side effects. A medication one person tolerates well can send another person into a tailspin. This is true for over-the-counter sleep medications as well as prescription drugs. Some may even stimulate rather than depress the central nervous system.

➤ *Vest or waist restraints* may help but should be used cautiously. Some people adjust to them well; others fight them. Request assistance from your community-health nurse about the correct way to attach them to your loved one and to the bed. They need to be tied securely enough so your loved one won't escape and fall. Make certain you can untie them quickly in case of an emergency.

There are a variety of styles to choose from, available through home-care supply stores. Injuries related to restraints have resulted in new rulings for nursing homes; most nursing homes no longer use them at night and rely on careful monitoring instead.

➤ Consider hiring *home health-care workers* for the night shift to allow you to get some sleep. Use the skills of the substitute caregivers you hire. Remember, you are paying them. They shouldn't be sleeping on the job! Set up a plan with them or their agency that will include their responsibilities, for example, a morning routine of bathing, toileting, dressing, shaving, nail care, and so on.

Let them do the tasks you find difficult to do or that rob you of your needed energy. If your loved one is awake for large blocks of time in the night, some of these activities could be completed then, while you sleep.

Be aware that some people with Alzheimer's may get up, get dressed, wander around the house for an hour or so, then head for the nearest chair or sofa and promptly fall asleep. Don't worry too much about where they sleep or what they're wearing. The important thing is that they do sleep.

If, in spite of all your efforts, your loved one is still prone to wander nocturnally, you'll need to provide for safety. See chapter nine for more information about this subject.

Leaving Home

Bill Stewart looked out the kitchen door. The moon hung full, illuminating the path to the road. Helen, Bill's wife, was asleep. She'd locked the kitchen door, just as she always did, but tonight she'd forgotten to remove the key. Bill saw it, turned it, and then stepped out into the moonlight.

The town was seven miles north of their farm. Bill turned right at the gate and headed down the lonely country road.

The next morning a frantic Helen and two policemen found Bill curled up on a bench in the center of town. Sleeping.

Helen and Bill were certainly not alone in their nocturnal experience. People with Alzheimer's frequently wander aimlessly through their homes. Often they wander away from them. Night or day. Of all the bizarre behavior patterns of Alzheimer's sufferers, wandering away from home and getting lost is one of the most disturbing to caregivers.

My husband ran away from home several times. I remember one time when he said he was going to pick blackberries. He took his pail and ran off in the rain. My daughter and I went after him, but we lost him the woods and had to go back home and call the fire department.

After we called, we started searching again. We finally found him ourselves, up on the hill. He was soaking wet. And his pail was empty.

You see those geraniums there in the window? Well, one time when I got home from work my wife had taken off. I found a couple of cuttings of geraniums along the street and then I found more. I just kept picking up geranium cuttings until I found her. When we got home I put all the cuttings in water. The ones in the window are their descendants.

There were two places I usually thought to look for my wife. One was the church. The other was the grocery store. One day she wasn't at either of those places. I looked everywhere and finally I came home.

After I'd been home awhile I got a phone call from my neighbor. He said he'd seen my wife wandering around the bank parking lot, and he'd persuaded her to let him bring her home. When she was well she would never walk away like that. I don't know where she thought she was going. That parking lot is three miles away.

One day Dad ran off into the woods. I spent an hour and a half looking for him. I was about to call the sheriff when he came out of the woods by our house, and they called me.

You know, the feelings of guilt and embarrassment we suffered in the beginning were totally unnecessary. But we didn't know what was happening.

Finally I said to my mother, "This man is sick. It's nothing to be ashamed of. Let's tell everybody." So we started with the neighbors. I told them all, "If you see my father wandering, let me know immediately." It was a good thing we did that.

Wandering off is not confined to wandering away from home. Sometimes people with Alzheimer's wander away when they're on vacation.

Three years ago my family was at a museum up north. In this museum you had to go in and out of different rooms to see the different exhibits.

We'd gone about two-thirds of the way around when we suddenly realized my wife wasn't with us. We figured she must have come out of one of the rooms and turned in the opposite direction from the rest of us.

We searched. We went all around the building and into other buildings. We looked everywhere. Finally we went out into the parking lot, and there she was. She'd gotten into the exit line and wandered out the gate.

When we came up to her she said to us, "Well, I found the camper, but I couldn't find the keys. If I had found them I'd have gone home."

And I think she would have. Or tried to. That was our first experience of wandering off. There have been many more since.

If your loved one strays away, you are faced with an emergency situation that could easily turn into tragedy. The phrase to remember is *don't panic*. The following strategies can help you cope.

▸ Don't spend time blaming yourself for your loved one's disappearance. Guilt won't help find anyone. If needed, call for assistance. Contact neighbors, friends, relatives, and the police to aid in the search. It's also good to let other people in the area know your loved one is lost. They may not be officially part of the search party, but they can be on the alert. Think about the obvious places your loved one might go—especially places familiar in the past—and share your information with the searchers.

▸ Search parties need a description of the person they're looking for. Have some recent color photographs at home. Also keep pictures of your loved one in the glove compartment of your car.

▸ Notify area hospital emergency rooms and nursing homes of your loved one's disappearance. If some Good Samaritan finds your loved one wandering down the road, they might go to a health-care facility.

▸ Your loved one should have an identification bracelet or necklace that says "memory impaired," "memory loss," or "Alzheimer's disease." It can also include name, address, and your phone number. If the person has a medical condition in addition to Alzheimer's, such as angina or diabetes, that information should be included along with allergies to any medications.

Identification (ID) jewelry can be purchased through your local pharmacy or home-care supply store and inexpensively engraved for you. There's a wide range of prices. Wallet-size ID cards are usually not a good substitute for an ID bracelet or necklace, because they can be easily lost or thrown away.

▸ Finding your loved one is only half the battle. Now you have to get him or her home. Chances are your loved one will be relieved to see you. She may be upset and know she's lost. On the other hand, you may not be seen as a rescuer but as someone to fend off or hide from.

Whatever the case, stay calm. Avoid running up, pulling on a sleeve, or trying to reason. Remind other rescuers that these techniques probably won't work. Instead, you might ask your loved one where he's going and offer to walk with him or take him with you. Most wanderers are looking for home. Home with you is where they really want to be.

If your loved one is always on the move, don't despair. With fore-sight, planning, and some practical strategies, we can maintain a relatively safe and secure environment for the perpetual or nocturnal wanderer. Looking for lost loved ones is a challenge most of us have to face at some point. It's a challenge we will meet when that point comes.

Chapter 8

Baffling Behaviors

My mother used to take me visiting with her a lot when I was a child. Occasionally we'd go to the homes of relatives who had knick-knacks and glassware lying around on tables and shelves, just waiting to be knocked off. But my mother had trained me well. I always walked around with my hands either behind my back or in my pockets. So did she!

When Mom developed Alzheimer's, she acted just the opposite, reaching out and touching everything in sight. Sometimes she took the things she touched.

Mom usually went grocery shopping with me. I would push her ahead of me in her portable wheelchair and pull the grocery cart behind us. When our shopping was completed, I carefully checked her pockets and the sleeves of her sweater before checking out. Mom had a tendency, often when I was busy looking in the frozen food section, to reach out and touch the assortment of packaged cakes and cookies in the middle of the aisle. If a package was small, colorful, and looked good to eat, my mother might pocket it for future consumption.

Hoarding

People with Alzheimer's are a little like pirates; they love to "rummage, pillage and hoard."[1] Then they may pocket the loot (food, shoes, neckties, jewelry, and so forth) and stash it away in a hiding place that they alone seem to know about.

In a nursing home where I occasionally work, one resident has a habit of wandering into other people's rooms and rummaging through their drawers, collecting things to "take home." I sometimes find her exiting a room carrying a shoe, a box of Kleenex, or underwear. Asking her to give up these items is like asking a toddler to relinquish a favorite toy. "No" is always the answer, accompanied by a set jaw and an even firmer grip on the pilfered items.

I'm usually able to retrieve them, though, if I offer to trade. The trade might take the form of a cookie, a cracker, a glass of milk, or a magazine. Sometimes it takes several trades to accomplish the task, but it works and we both wind up happy. (I found this also worked with another resident who had a habit of "stealing" the fire extinguisher!)

> It got to the point where everybody was "stealing" Dad's stuff. He thought people were coming in the house and hiding things from him, but he was really the one who was doing the hiding.
>
> My father was forever losing his toolbox. It was his prized possession, so he would hide it—and then forget where he hid it. One of his favorite hiding places was under the china closet in the living room. But sometimes the toolbox wound up under the bed or down in the cellar.
>
> He'd say to my mother, "Where are my tools? What did you do with them?" And, to keep the peace, my mother would have to go with him and search for them.

> There was this terrible odor coming from my mother's room. The aides finally figured it out. Mom had tucked away a chicken leg in the drawer of her bedside stand.

How do we solve the problem of taking and losing things? Asking "Where did you hide it this time?" doesn't usually work. There are gentle, loving, and practical ways to discover where your wife stashed the family jewels or where your father hid the house keys.

➤ Have a place only you know about to put car keys, cash, and other irreplaceable items. Make small and easily lost articles more visible by attaching them to larger and more colorful things, like key rings. Be sure you have duplicates of whatever can be duplicated.

➤ Put mail and other important papers out of reach and out of sight. Many Alzheimer's sufferers don't just hide things, they also rip them up.

➤ Check the contents of wastebaskets before throwing out the trash.

➤ Lock the bathroom door if your loved one has a tendency to flush away valuables.

➤ You may need to lock inner doors, closets, and dresser drawers. This not only protects other people's valuables but also eliminates hiding places.

➤ Think of some of the not-so-obvious places where your loved one might hide things, if you're truly stumped. Check the folds of chairs and sofas. Examine pocketbooks or wallets. Look in bowls and dishes in the kitchen.

➤ If your loved one tends to hoard valuable things, use substitutes. Buy some cheap costume jewelry and store your good stuff in a place your loved one isn't likely to look. If he or she stashes away food that spoils, make packages of crackers available. Nibbling at various times during the day or night may be the result of legitimate hunger. Provide for this need.

➤ Keep a "rummage box" that can be used as a substitute when your loved one starts rummaging through dresser drawers.

➤ Don't expect your loved one to remember the hiding places of the car keys or the mail. Asking or demanding will only create a stressful situation. Simply expect to join in the search from time to time.

Rummaging, pillaging, hiding, and hoarding are behaviors common to people with Alzheimer's. The reasons are unclear, but the need for security may be an underlying factor. Creating a secure environment is a challenge we all face as we care for our loved ones. It is a challenge that can try our patience. It can also make us more tolerant and sensitive people.

Losing Control

Difficulties with bladder and bowel elimination usually become a problem as Alzheimer's progresses. Incontinence of urine and stool occurs frequently and can present a real physical and emotional dilemma for the unprepared caregiver. Incontinence can also be embarrassing. It requires us to keep our sense of humor and sense of perspective.

> I remember the day my wife had a bowel movement in the grocery store. I was mortified. But they were so good to us. One young store clerk came up behind us and rolled up the rug. Luckily my wife did it in the right spot.

> My mother was incontinent once right in the bank. I was making a deposit and when I turned around, there she was, taking off her wet diapers over by the window. I ran over, grabbed the diapers, stuffed them in my pocketbook, and got her out of there. Fast.
>
> Just last week I saw a two-year-old in a store downtown do the same thing. Her mother reacted the same way I did. I think you need a sense of humor in this business.

> My husband is totally incontinent now and has been for quite a while. His urologist told me that one of the things I could expect eventually was lack of control of bowels and bladder. The bad thing about it was that my husband sometimes went

in back of the barn and shed his clothes, including his diapers. He'd throw the wet or soiled diapers aside and then put his clothes back on. I think there's quite a pile of diapers out in back of the barn, in the raspberry bushes.

In addition to getting rid of our embarrassment, we need to lose the notion that toileting is a very personal, very private affair. Sooner or later we'll have to get involved in this aspect of our loved one's care.

The biggest problem I had was when my wife first became incontinent. She'd wet the bed at night and I decided, well, I'll just have to get her up. It was tough because she was a sound sleeper and resisted me. Often before I could get her to the toilet she'd urinate on the floor. It used to make me so mad because I didn't understand what was happening.

Finally I decided there was just no sense trying to get her up and getting mad. It didn't do her any good and it didn't do me any good. So I got some disposable adult diapers, a rubber sheet, and some smaller sheets they call draw sheets, and I put them on the bed. If she was swimming in the morning, that was all right. I just had extra laundry to do.

The following are suggestions for preventing and dealing with incontinence, should it occur, as well as other aspects of bladder and bowel management.

➤ If incontinence of urine becomes a problem at any stage of Alzheimer's disease, don't assume it's due to the Alzheimer's process. This is especially true if symptoms appear suddenly. There may be an underlying medical problem, such as a urinary tract infection (UTI). Initially it's wise to talk to your doctor. A simple urine test may be recommended to see if there's an infection that could easily be treated with an antibiotic. Untreated urinary tract infections can worsen any incontinence related to Alzheimer's.

Women are more prone than men to develop UTIs because it is easier for infectious agents to move up and into the female bladder. Symptoms of urinary tract infections and more severe kidney infections can include any or all of the following:

- frequent urge to urinate
- urinating in small amounts
- difficulty starting to urinate
- burning, pain, or stinging on urination
- foul-smelling urine
- cloudy, blood-tinged, or mucus-tinged urine
- abdominal pain or discomfort
- fever and chills
- nausea and vomiting
- back pain
- increased confusion

➤ Some medications can contribute to urinary incontinence—water pills or diuretics, for example. It's usually best to give these early in the morning to prevent incontinence at night.

Some tranquilizers and sedatives can have the opposite effect and result in urine retention that, if unnoticed and untreated, can be a serious, even life-threatening problem. The medication haloperidol (Haldol), frequently prescribed for people with Alzheimer's, is one notable example. A pharmacist is usually a good source of information about drug side effects.

If your loved ones are on medication that can cause urinary side effects, you need to carefully observe their toileting habits.

➤ Anticipate accidents. Become aware of mannerisms that may indicate a need to urinate or have a bowel movement.

➤ Minimize accidents by having your loved one cut down on fluid intake, especially tea and coffee, several hours before bedtime. Fluids should not usually be limited during the day, however, except for other medical reasons. Adequate fluid intake is essential for proper hydration and can also help prevent urinary tract infections and constipation.

If in doubt, check with your physician. The necessary amount of fluid may vary from person to person. Dehydration as well as overhydration can contribute to confusion.

➤ Toilet at regular intervals—every two to three hours, before or after meals, and just prior to retiring. Do this even if your loved one wears an adult diaper or brief. Through regular toileting, a habit pattern can form that may keep him or her dry throughout the day and night. It's definitely worth your effort and a little trial and error.

➤ Minimize the distance from bedroom to bathroom. Consider the use of a bedside commode.

➤ Think about using an adult diaper or brief or, for minimal incontinence and dribbling, a sanitary pad or baby diaper worn inside the underwear.

There are many different brands of briefs available through home-care supply stores and pharmacies. Costs vary. Some people's skin may be sensitive to some brands. You may need to experiment if your loved one develops a rash.

Ask your community-health nurse or home-care supply dealer for tips on how to put the diapers on when a person is lying down or standing up. Rubber pants are also available in adult sizes.

Adult briefs may help your loved one (and you) feel more secure when out and about, though there is often an understandable initial reaction to "needing to be diapered again, like a baby," as one caregiver put it. If your loved one does not take them off at night, adult briefs may help you both get a good night's rest. Be sensitive, though, to your loved one's feelings of shame, embarrassment, and loss of self-esteem.

➤ Skin tissue is very sensitive to urine and can break down quickly if not kept clean and dry. Soap and water is all you need. Avoid perfumed powders; they can contribute to UTIs. Cornstarch may be an alternative if perspiration around skin folds in the abdomen and groin area is a problem.

As with urine, stool on the skin can result in skin breakdown and even urinary tract infections. If you need to assist your loved one with hygiene, wipe and wash well, wiping and/or washing from front (urinary opening) to back (rectal area).

➤ Protect the bed with a waterproof mattress cover. A large sheet of plastic or an old shower curtain also works well. Disposable or cloth bed pads with waterproof backing are available and can cut down on laundry. Simple draw sheets (smaller pieces of sheeting) or pillowcases with a piece of plastic inside may also work well and are inexpensive alternatives.

To control odors from urine, wash mattress covers regularly with soap and water, and spray with a disinfectant.

➤ Indwelling catheters are usually not recommended for the management of incontinence because they can easily contribute to infections and are often pulled out by people with dementia. External catheters that fit like condoms may, however, be useful for some men who experience incontinence at night and are heavy sleepers.

➤ If urinary retention and difficulty starting a urine stream are problems, try running water in the sink or tub when your loved one is on the toilet.

Bowel habits differ from person to person. Some people move their bowels daily, others every two to three days. A person with dementia may have difficulty keeping a normal schedule for a variety of reasons related to the disease process, diet, lack of exercise, various medications, and so on. If diarrhea is a problem, it may be related to a stomach upset or injudicious use of laxatives.

A more frequently occurring problem is constipation. Signs of constipation include pain in the abdominal or rectal area, irregular and infrequent bowel movements, discomfort or pain when having a bowel movement, diarrhea or liquid leakage around a hard, impacted stool, and headaches.

The best way to prevent constipation is through a diet adequate in liquids, fiber, and bulk. Breakfast is often the best meal for adding fiber. You might try sprinkling bran on hot cereal or serving a high fiber cereal. (A fiber cereal mixed with yogurt and fruit is a nutritious way to increase fiber and bulk.) Substitute whole-grain breads for white. Add more raw fruits and vegetables to your loved one's menu.

➤ Lack of exercise can contribute to constipation. Remember the therapeutic value of walking.

➤ Constipation is also a frequent side effect of some medications, especially those prescribed for pain. Ask your pharmacist. You may need to switch to another type of pain reliever if the problem persists.

➤ If diet and exercise fail to work, consider the use of stool softeners, either prescription or over-the-counter. Some are available in liquid or powder form.

    Overuse of laxatives such as milk of magnesia may lead to bowel inactivity. Avoid them, if possible.

➤ Suppositories may help some people. They are available in mild over-the-counter forms or by prescription. Drugstores also carry various name-brand and generic-brand enemas that are relatively easy to administer and may need to be used on occasion. If you have any questions about how to give an enema, check with your community-health nurse.

Losing control can be an embarrassment for the Alzheimer's sufferer and a management problem for the caregiver. But we need to remember that it is a *manageable* problem, a problem that can be minimized with the proper resources and our resourcefulness.

Managing Mealtimes

Mealtimes usually include fun and fellowship as well as food. But when you're caring for a person with Alzheimer's, mealtimes can be times of frustration. Eating isn't always a sit-down occasion.

My father wouldn't sit down for his meals. He decided he'd rather stand. He'd say, "I gotta do this" and "I gotta do that," and then he'd eat a little and run around the house. He was extremely hyper.

Judgment and coordination are sometimes affected, and the memory for eating and perhaps even for swallowing becomes impaired for some people.

My brother can't always judge where his food is. We have to put it in his hand. He does a lot better with finger food, with things he can feel. Silverware seems too hard for him to manage, and I think he has trouble feeling it because it's so thin. He eats sandwiches, bananas, cheese, things like that.

My mother sits down at the table but then can't remember how to eat, or what to do with her fork or spoon. I usually have to get her started, and sometimes the old memory seems to come back and kick in. At other times it doesn't, and I have to feed her an entire meal.

It got so it took forever for my wife to eat. It took over an hour for lunch. Sometimes she'd chew something for ten minutes before she'd swallow it.

You know how you do with a baby sometimes? You stroke the baby's throat? That's what I'd do with my wife. I'd say, "Come on, now. Swallow, swallow, swallow." And then, when she was ready, she'd swallow.

Sometimes a person may refuse to eat. At other times he or she will eat everything in sight.

My husband eats everything he can get his hands on, but he doesn't gain any weight. He runs it off the rest of the time.

My wife seemed to lose her appetite one day and refused to eat. Now it's a hard job to get anything down her. I know she's depressed, too, and that accounts for some of it.

People with Alzheimer's, particularly in the later stages, are prone to respiratory infections like pneumonia. These may be precipitated by choking on food.

Some people with Alzheimer's have trouble swallowing, and instead of food going down their esophagus it goes down their windpipe. I think that's what happened to my wife. She got pneumonia after an episode of choking one day at the nursing home.

The following suggestions may help make mealtimes more manageable at various stages in the disease.

➤ Decrease stimulation in the environment. Maintain a calm atmosphere at mealtimes. Play quiet music instead of loud television shows. Consider subdued lighting instead of a bright glare.

➤ In meal planning, choose from the basic four food groups for a well-rounded diet. These include for a day:

- Protein. Two to three servings of the following: meat, poultry, fish, cheese, eggs, dried beans, peas, nuts.
- Carbohydrates. Four servings of bread, cereal, potatoes. Whole-grain breads are best.
- Dairy. Two or more cups of milk or milk products such as ice cream, cottage cheese, yogurt.
- Fruits and vegetables. Four or more servings including dark green or deep yellow vegetables, tomatoes, and citrus fruits.

Focus on familiar foods your loved one has always liked. Many finger foods, including sandwiches, cheese, fruits, and vegetables, can meet the "basic four" requirements and also meet the needs of a person who is always on the go.

➤ Small, frequent meals or snacks may be more acceptable than large, sit-down dinners three times a day.

➤ To increase nutrition for the finicky eater, leave snacks around or add the following supplements during the day:

- milk shakes (add ice cream, vanilla, sweetener, flavoring, an egg to a glass of milk)
- puddings, custards, yogurt
- instant breakfast drinks (also add them to milk shakes)

➤ If swallowing or chewing becomes a problem, try grinding or blending foods. This is preferable to canned baby foods and enables you to cook the same meal for the whole family. A food processor, blender, or small grinder will work well. Thick liquids are often swallowed more easily than thinner liquids. Try cream soups for easier swallowing and added nourishment.

➤ Try the following steps for alleviating coordination problems:

- Substitute bowls for plates, or consider using a plate guard to minimize accidental spilling.
- Switch to unbreakable dishes.
- Build up utensil handles to make them easier to feel and hold.
- Offer only one food at a time if your loved one has difficulty making choices.

➤ If you must feed your loved one, consider the following:

- Sit, don't stand, when feeding. Maintain eye contact.
- Converse naturally, but don't encourage a lot of talking or laughter that could contribute to choking.

- Spoons often work better than forks for feeding.
- Approach your loved one directly, not from the side. Feed him or her using a gentle, downward pressure on the center of the tongue.
- If there is any weakness or paralysis related to a stroke or multi-infarct dementia, feed on the unaffected side to make chewing and swallowing easier.
- Be sensitive to the temperature of foods, especially when foods are microwaved. Your loved one may not be able to communicate discomfort.
- Take your time. Don't rush. You may need to encourage your loved one to swallow after each bite or make sure food isn't being squirreled away in ever-bulging cheeks.

➤ As an added safety precaution, learn the Heimlich, or abdominal-thrust, maneuver. This is a relatively simple procedure that has saved thousands of lives. It is something all of us should know, with or without a loved one with Alzheimer's.

Hospitals and nursing homes always teach their employees this procedure. You might be able to attend a class (usually about an hour in length) by calling their in-service coordinator and explaining your need. If you can't attend a class or demonstration, refer to a first-aid book.

Remember that eating out doesn't have to stop when your loved one has Alzheimer's. Enjoying a meal with a loved one at home or away is one of those things that can still be a part of life.

I used to take my wife to the nutrition center run by the office on aging in our town. It was good for us both. It got me out and provided her with more stimulation than she had at home. We made a lot of friends there too.

I take my husband out to eat quite a lot. He sometimes spills things, and occasionally I have to feed him. I have a couple of places we go pretty regularly, usually when it's not very crowded. They all know us and the waitresses are great. You don't have to stop doing things you've always enjoyed just because you have Alzheimer's, you know.

Sexual Disinhibitions

My husband undresses himself a lot in the nursing home, right in the middle of the dining room. Sometimes he asks the other residents and even the aides if they will go to bed with him. If he were in his right mind he'd be humiliated.

My sister was always a very shy, withdrawn person but she isn't anymore. You should hear the language that comes out of her mouth when they try to give her a shower. She also tries to grab people if they get too close to her—and not in very acceptable places.

Loss of impulse control, causing a person to engage in inappropriate sexual behavior of which they are not aware of because of their state of disorientation, is not common to most Alzheimer's sufferers. But when it does occur it can be particularly distressing to the family caregiver at home. If their loved one is in a nursing care facility, family members need to know their loved one will be treated with dignity and respect and not made fun of or be treated with contempt.

Often behavior that may appear sexual in nature may be caused for various other reasons. For example, the person who wanders around partially clothed or with a blouse unbuttoned or pants unzipped may have simply forgotton how to dress themselves. Due to the degree of their dementia, they may be totally unaware of their state of undress.

A calm, gentle, but firm approach to reorient a person back to their bedroom or a bathroom where you can assist them in redressing is often all that is needed to solve the problem. In nursing homes, trying to redress a person in a busy hall or noisy dining area often will precipitate a catastrophic reaction. The person may think they are being molested; not a few persons with Alzheimer's have cried "rape" when caregivers with good intentions have tried to help them.

If zippers on pants are continually becoming unzipped and shirts and blouses unbuttoned, switch to pull-on pants and pull-over shirts and sweaters. Dresses that zip in the back are better for women who have a tendency to fidget with their clothes.

Masturbation may also occur in public places and may be engaged in simply because it feels good to the brain-damaged person. Distraction will often work if the person's attention can be redirected to something else to hold or touch. Masturbation can also be prompted by poor genital hygiene, or itching related to a urinary tract infection that prompts rubbing the genital area for relief. Carefully assess possible underlying physical reasons for this behavior, such as the adequacy of hygiene.

Sexual overtures, or what are interpreted as sexual overtures, may be made in nursing home or hospital settings to other residents, patients, visitors, and staff members. Often the person with dementia will simply mistake the other people for a beloved spouse and treat them accordingly. They may climb into bed with another resident of the opposite sex, simply because they have always slept with a spouse and have no idea that this is not their own room or their own bed. A gentle but firm approach can guide the person with dementia back to their own room and bed; the rights of other residents need to be protected, but the affectional and relationship needs for closeness and companionship of the person with dementia should also be addressed.

The impact of Alzheimer's on the marital relationship, including all the varying dimensions of sexuality and intimacy, can be devastating for caregivers. As Lore Wright, in *Alzheimer's Disease and Marriage* notes, Robert Browning's poem that includes the familiar lines, "Grow old along with me! The best is yet to be . . ." rings hollow for many couples when a spouse has Alzheimer's.[2]

Sensitive marital counseling with a professional very familiar with Alzheimer's disease may be needed. Other caregiving spouses can also be supportive and may welcome the opportunity to share concerns and strategies with others in similar situations. A number of helpful references are included in appendix A for married couples in need of additional support and information.

Chapter 9

The Struggle for Safety

Safety is always an issue with older people, especially those living alone and in frail health. Add dementia, and safety becomes an all-consuming concern that can spell catastrophe. Preventive measures have to be taken. And fortunately, there are many things we can do to ensure our loved ones' safety, as well as our own.

Taking Away the Car Keys

Most of us drive by habit. If the way is familiar, we're often unaware of the various roads we pass or the towns we drive through. Yet if the sudden and unexpected should occur, all our senses go on the alert. We are usually able to make a quick judgment, respond appropriately, and avoid an accident.

This may not be the case, though, with Alzheimer's sufferers, who may be unable to respond quickly or logically to a sudden, unexpected event. Although vision may remain intact and hearing unaffected, the ability to make decisions about what they are seeing and hearing—and even where they are going—is progressively impaired.[1]

> One day my husband turned around, right in the middle of the road. We were on Main Street in the city at the time. The next thing I knew, we were headed up the one-way ramp—going the wrong way—on the expressway. I said to myself, "This is it. I can't cope with this any longer."

I used to pray every day for other drivers because my father was a maniac on the road. He had been an excellent mechanic and driver, but as his disease progressed he became careless and dangerous. He gave me a ride one day that was enough to make my hair turn white. It was the most awful experience of my life.

Our identity is partly defined for us by the things we do, particularly the things we do well. Driving is something most of us, especially men, are expected to do and do well.

Being told you cannot drive, that you are no longer safe on the road, can be a tremendous blow to a person's ego. Regardless of the degree of memory impairment, a person still responds on a feeling level when identity is threatened. People with Alzheimer's often won't relinquish the wheel voluntarily.

My husband's driving drove me crazy, but I couldn't convince him to stop. You'd think he'd been on a ten-day drinking binge the way he acted behind the wheel.

I'd holler, I'd scream, I'd stamp my feet. I even threatened to leave him once. It didn't make any difference. He kept insisting he could drive just fine.

My car was being fixed the day we had our family reunion. After the reunion Dad took me to the garage and he started tailgating a motorcycle driver. He was only about two feet ahead of us and the poor guy couldn't go any faster. He was behind another car, sandwiched in by my father.

I said, "Don't you think you're a little close?"

He just glared at me and said, "Oh, it's all right." He could never understand that his judgment was wrong.

Convincing a loved one to stop driving may be the most difficult thing we'll ever have to do as caregivers. But it must be done; usually the sooner, the better.

How soon is *soon?* We can take our cues from our loved ones. If there are obvious impairments in other areas of their behavior that involve judgment, concentration, and coordination, as well as time, place, and person orientation, the ability to drive safely also will be impaired. It will only worsen.

The following strategies may be helpful:

➤ Begin with a gentle person-to-person approach. You may find yourself pleasantly surprised. Your loved one may consider it a relief not to have to drive. Don't assume he or she wants to continue driving.

➤ Many caregivers find that it helps to pray before talking with the loved one. Avoid judging or criticizing driving skills. Instead, consider the person's feelings and empathize. It should be easy: you know how you'd feel if you were in a similar position. Focus on the safety issues involved.

➤ One caregiver told me, "I hid my husband's glasses. I hid the car keys. I removed the distributor cap. I disconnected the starter wire. Alzheimer's makes you real sneaky."

You may have to do any or all of these things at some point if your loved one insists on driving, though perhaps a better solution is to visibly remove the object of the temptation. If you don't drive, this shouldn't be a problem. If you do, check with a neighbor or nearby garage about keeping your vehicle for your use only.

➤ Ask your physician to speak with your loved one or write a letter or a "prescription" stating he or she can no longer drive.

The doctor bailed me out and it worked just fine. He took my husband into his office, sat him down and said, "George, how many years have you been driving? Don't you think it would be a good idea if you sat in the passenger seat for a while and let your wife do the driving for you both?"

I guess it must have been the voice of authority. I never had to speak about it to my husband again. He just quit driving.

My father was always a respecter of the law regarding his driver's license. He knew you couldn't get in the car without it. He would always say, "Have I got my license?"

We finally convinced the doctor that Dad was dangerous on the road. The doctor wrote him a letter stating he could no longer drive. When we got the letter, my dad gave my mother his license. He just voluntarily handed it over. He seemed to respect the doctor's authority.

Someone else may have the voice of authority in your loved one's life—your doctor, the insurance agent, a lawyer, or the Department of Motor Vehicles. If this is the case, enlist their help. Stress the importance of safety for both your loved one and other people. If necessary, your physician can request a retesting by the Department of Motor Vehicles. Licenses can be suspended. Rules vary from state to state, so consult your local motor vehicle department for information.

➤ If your loved one lives alone but still has a desire to get out and about, you'll need to provide for transportation that is safe. Sharing the responsibility with family members, friends, and neighbors can ease the burden. Taxi services or a senior-citizen bus or van may be an economical alternative in some areas.

Inquire about transportation options through your area office of aging or through community organizations that serve the elderly. Regular routes that transport people to and from nutrition sites, for example, might help meet your loved one's need for socialization and nutrition, as well as the need to be "on the go." Billing can usually be arranged.

If you hire home-care workers and feel it is safe for your loved one to ride in a car, consider employing at least one aide who is willing to drive and is appropriately licensed and insured. If you hire through an agency, check its transportation policies. Many agencies will not allow aides to transport but may forget to tell you this when you apply for help.

➤ You may never have thought of yourself as adventurous. A spouse with Alzheimer's may change all that, particularly if getting out and going places is important to you.

If you don't drive and want to learn, check with your local high school or vocational school about driver education classes. Learning to drive at age fifty-five or sixty is not impossible or impractical. In fact, it may be the best gift you can give yourself both now and for the future.

➤ Finally, "treat" your loved one with chauffeuring. Say, "It's time you relaxed and enjoyed the view," as one caregiver successfully told her spouse. You may discover that you both will actually enjoy yourselves and the scenery for the first time in months.

Remember, driving is a learned activity that quickly becomes unlearned. It's therefore a dangerous activity for someone with Alzheimer's. Driving is also a habit. Like all habits, if it's not practiced, it soon fades away. It's important that it fades before any serious or tragic injuries occur.

Home Safety

> We no longer wanted to leave my mother alone, not for even a little while. We were always afraid she'd start a fire with her smoking. She'd light the wrong end of the cigarette sometimes and try to put it in her mouth. She'd also drop cigarettes when they were lit or stuff them in the corners of the couch to put them out. She had a plastic tablecloth on the kitchen table that was covered with cigarette burns.

> We had a wood stove in the garage, and one day we found my father trying to light it with a propane torch. We took the torch away. Anything we thought might be dangerous we took away.
> One day we found Dad turning on the fire on the gas stove. Dad had cut up a drop light with a long cord, and was trying to weld it together again with the flames of the stove. When I

tried to take it away from him, he bawled me out for buying something "cheap and inferior." He told me it was no good. All I can say is, you have to be alert!

Safety in and around the house is always a concern for the older person, especially the older person who lives alone or who is confused or disoriented. What is a safety hazard for one person may not be a hazard for another. A flat iron may present no problem to a man who has never ironed in his life, and an older woman may not feel the urge to rummage through her husband's toolbox.

We don't have to totally reconstruct our houses, but we do have to know our loved one's habits. We have to be alert. Decide what are potential hazards for your loved one, remembering that these may change as the disease progresses. Here are some specific situations to consider:

1. *Prevent burns from fire, water, and electricity.*

➤ Lock up electrical equipment such as hair dryers and electric shavers if there is danger of your loved one's plugging them in and dropping them in the sink or tub.

➤ Turn down the temperature of your water heater if your loved one can no longer judge hot from cold.

➤ Monitor smoking by keeping matches and lighters in your possession.

Many caregivers have found that breaking a lifelong habit of smoking was unexpectedly easy for someone with Alzheimer's. Cigarettes, cigars, and pipes that are out of sight may quickly fade out of mind as well.

➤ Remove knobs from your gas stove or turn off the shut-off valve at night if your loved one wanders and tries to cook.

➤ Unplug electrical appliances in the kitchen. Consider coverings for electrical outlets.

➤ Have a fire extinguisher in your kitchen that can be used for all types of fires. Install smoke detectors in appropriate places and test them regularly.

➤ Plan escape routes from the various rooms in your house in case there is ever a need to evacuate.

2. *Minimize cuts and bruises.*

➤ Lock up knives, power tools, and other sharp objects.

➤ Pad the corners of sharp pieces of furniture.

➤ Check glassware and other dishes periodically for cracks.

3. *Avoid accidental poisoning.*

➤ Keep medications in a safe, dry place, not in a kitchen cabinet or the bathroom medicine closet. If necessary, lock them up.

➤ Lock up poisonous cleaning supplies or store them in inaccessible places.

➤ Keep the phone number of the poison control center next to your phone.

➤ Invest in a first-aid kit for poisoning that will include syrup of ipecac and activated charcoal. Vomiting should be induced for some, but not all, poisonous substances. Container labels and the poison control center can tell you the difference.

Be aware of the signs of poisoning, which may include any of the following:

- nausea, vomiting, diarrhea
- severe abdominal pain, cramping
- slow breathing and slow pulse
- profuse sweating or salivation

- obvious burns or stains around the mouth
- odors on the breath, such as kerosene or turpentine
- unconsciousness
- convulsions

4. Decrease the danger of falls.

Falls become more problematic as Alzheimer's disease progresses and areas of the brain which control muscles and coordination are affected. The following tips can help accident-proof your home against falls.

➤ Avoid high-gloss waxing of linoleum or wood floors.

➤ Eliminate loose throw rugs or else anchor them firmly, especially in the bathroom.

➤ Make sure all electrical and phone cords are outside traffic areas.

➤ Get rid of chairs that tip over easily. Solid and familiar furniture, strategically placed, can be an ambulation aid.

➤ Clear away clutter, especially on stairs.

➤ Remove doorway thresholds and replace them with flat stripping.

➤ Put locks at the top or bottom of cellar and exit doors. Lock windows if necessary or disguise them with drapes. Alarms can also be installed on windows and doors.

➤ Shelve frequently used items in easily reached places.

➤ Light up nocturnal trips from bedroom to bathroom with a 25-watt soft-light bulb, or consider night-lights in various rooms.

➤ Install safety grab bars in areas around toilet, tub, and shower. Use suction mats or nonslip tub strips in tub and shower.

► Periodically check the soles and heels of shoes and slippers for wear. Thin, worn soles can be slippery.

► Avoid long hems and trailing sleeves in your loved one's nightwear.

► Falls most frequently occur on the top or bottom stair step. Paint both steps in contrasting colors or use bright paint strips. Make certain stair railings are solid and secure. Block the bottom and top of the stairwell with a sturdy gate if needed.

► Outside, make sure your entryway is well lit, pool areas are well secured, and sidewalks are in good repair.

► If your loved one needs help walking, consider purchasing a cane or walker. Another possibility is an ambulation or walking belt. (This can also be used to help get a person in and out of a chair or bed with minimal effort on the part of the caregiver.) Talk with your loved one's physician or call the therapy department in your local hospital for instructions on how to use one or, better yet, ask for a home demonstration through your county nursing agency. Such agencies usually have a physical therapist who can help caregivers learn to use assistive devices.

5. *Get help if needed.*
If your loved one should fall, don't panic. Be especially careful if you attempt to break a loved one's fall. Take time to assess the situation. It may be an emergency, but chances are it is not life-threatening.

► If for any reason you suspect a fracture or head injury, *do not attempt to move your loved one.* Simply make him or her as comfortable as possible. Use a blanket to prevent chilling, and use a rolled up blanket or pillow to support an injured limb. Then call the emergency squad for help. Don't ask friends or neighbors to help you move your loved one to a more comfortable position; this could cause further damage to a fractured limb.

Some signs of a fracture include:

- pain or tenderness in the injured area that increases with pressure or movement
- deformity (for example, a fractured hip may cause one leg to appear shorter and to rotate outward)
- swelling (not always immediate)
- discoloration or bruising
- exposed bone ends that have broken through the skin
- possible shock (cold, pale, clammy skin; rapid pulse; shallow breathing)

If you don't suspect a fracture, but are not sure you can help your loved one on your own, get help. Call a neighbor or the police.

Falling can be a symptom of other problems, such as medication side effects, poor vision, small strokes, low blood pressure, and so on. A physical exam may be in order if you notice any obvious and sudden changes in your loved one's ability to navigate around the house.

Educate Yourself and Be Prepared

Investing in a good family first-aid book can help you feel more confident if an emergency should arise. You might also want to purchase a first-aid kit or have the following supplies on hand:

- adhesive bandages
- large and small sterile gauze dressings
- soft gauze roller bandages
- adhesive or paper tape
- scissors
- a triangular bandage
- a poison antidote (syrup of ipecac, activated charcoal)
- ice packs you can keep in the freezer

Home safety for the person with Alzheimer's is much the same as home safety for anyone else: a little common sense, a little foresight into possible hazards, and a little knowledge of what to do and when to do it goes a long way.

When the Emergency Is You

"In the event of an emergency," I told one of the home-care aides I'd hired, "I can be reached at my work phone number."

"Fine," she said. "But what if the emergency is *you?* What if you get hit by a bus or your car lands in a ditch? What do I do with your mother?"

I had never really thought about it.

As caregivers of loved ones with Alzheimer's, we hope and pray *we* won't ever wind up as a medical or surgical emergency, but that possibility is always present. Contrary to what most of us would like to believe, we're not immune from our own disasters or even deaths.

There's a good motto for caregivers who find themselves thinking about their own mortality: Be prepared.

1. Have emergency numbers handy.

If aides care for your loved one in your home while you are away, the substitute caregivers should know how to reach you. Provide them with a list of emergency phone numbers that might include:

- relative(s), friend(s), neighbor(s)
- your primary physician; your loved one's physician
- the hospital emergency room
- ambulance or emergency squad
- police
- fire department
- poison control center

Substitute caregivers need to know who will be responsible for your loved one should you suddenly become incapacitated. Who, specifically, should they call?

They should also have the county adult protective service number in case no one on their list can be contacted and emergency caregiving arrangements need to be made.

Keep a list of emergency numbers at home even if you don't hire help. It will be available in times of need.

If your loved one stays at a day-care center, you will need to tell the staff where you can be reached and provide information about what to do if something should happen to you.

2. Prepare emergency-care notebooks.

Some caregivers keep a notebook of all the vital information someone else would need in order to assume caregiving responsibilities in case of an emergency.

Setting aside a few hours to organize such a notebook will be well worth the effort and can contribute to your peace of mind. A notebook will prove an invaluable resource if a substitute caregiver comes into your home to care for your loved one. It can also benefit professional and paraprofessional caregivers in an adult home or nursing home setting if your loved one needs alternative living arrangements. Your notebook might include some of the following information:

➤ *Daily routine.* If your loved one has a daily routine, it's wise to include this in as much detail as possible. For example, "7:00— Usually wakes up. 7:15—Help out of bed to bedside commode. 7:30—Give sponge bath and dress." What can your loved one do independently? What do you have to help with?

➤ *Nutritional needs.* What are your loved one's eating habits and problems? Are there favorite foods? Dislikes? Allergies? Is there a favorite area to eat in? Any special dishes or utensils? Can your loved one feed himself or herself? Does he or she snack during the day?

➤ *Sleep patterns.* What is your loved one's normal bedtime routine? Are naps common? If nighttime wandering is a problem, what do you do to manage this behavior?

▶ *Toileting concerns.* If there's a special toileting routine to prevent or control incontinence, include details for both bladder and bowel habits.

▶ *Medications.* What medications does your loved one take? Include the name of each drug, dosage, and time to be taken. Does your loved one swallow pills without difficulty, or do pills have to be crushed and given in food or drink?

▶ *Special behavior problems.* If there are any specific problems, such as wandering or "sundowning," include these. (See chapter six for additional examples.)

▶ *Social history.* Jot down anything that will make communication with your loved one easier—the name he or she likes to be called, information about likes, dislikes, interests, occupation. Help the substitute caregiver know your loved one as a person to relate to, not a problem to solve.

Watching Over Your Loved One

It is impossible to prepare for every calamity that might occur in our lives as caregivers. But several additional safety measures can provide important safeguards against the unknown.

For example, if your own health is frail, consider installing an emergency response unit at home that can be attached to your telephone. Commonly known as "life-lines," these units connect your home phone to a local hospital emergency room and can be activated at the press of a button (usually carried or worn).

Identification jewelry can be especially vital for your loved one should the two of you be involved in an accident or should you suddenly become ill.

If you suddenly need to go to the hospital and there is no time to make emergency arrangements, insist that your loved one go with you. Have the hospital social worker notified en route or upon arrival so special arrangements can be made for his or her care. Carry emergency numbers with you in a wallet or purse. It is often wise planning to arrange for someone to have power of attorney over you as well as over your loved one, in case you become incapacitated. Talk with your lawyer about this.

It's never pleasant to think of our own ill health, but denial of the possibility is guaranteed to bring future grief should we suddenly become dependent.

Plan ahead. Be prepared.

Part Three

CARING FOR YOURSELF

*The deepest lessons come out of the deepest
waters and the hottest fires.*

Elisabeth Elliot, *A Path Through Suffering*

Chapter 10

People Who Help

I have always thought of myself as an active person. My solo lifestyle has meant a full-time job plus numerous activities outside the home. Moving back to New York to care for two older parents with health problems (my mother with Alzheimer's and my father diagnosed with cancer) threatened to change all that. I found myself calling out for help.

From a socioeconomic standpoint, my parents and I fell into what I consider a lower-middle income bracket. We were not poor enough to be eligible for any supplementary health programs offered by our county and not rich enough to afford many services either. Also, many services available in more metropolitan areas are simply not available in our predominantly rural area. I realized that creative and cost-effective measures were in order if I wanted to maintain my own emotional and physical health. Caregiving can take its toll on both.

A verse in the New Testament book of Galatians begins, "Carry each other's burdens" There are many burdens we can help each other carry. As caregivers, we need other people to help us. *We need to learn to lean.*

Leaning on others is not a sign of weakness. Admitting we need other people to help us occasionally can be a sign of strength—as well as a great relief. Allowing others to help us strengthens us for our caregiving responsibilities.

Help can come in many forms and from a surprising number of places. This section looks at a variety of support systems available to the caregiver and offers some suggestions for using them. Caregiving is hard, but it doesn't have to be an unbearable burden. There are many ways to lighten the load.

Support Groups

My mother wandered, never slept at night, and repeated the same words and phrases dozens of times a day. But it was my father who needed help most. Mother was well taken care of, but my dad suffered from frayed emotions, fatigue, and a flagging spirit. Dad needed a support group. And when I moved back to New York State to help him care for my mother, I found that I needed one too.

Shortly after I returned home, a letter in our newspaper gave the phone number for a local Alzheimer's support group. I called the number and talked with one of the support-group members for over an hour. She invited me to a meeting and encouraged me to take Mom to a physician who was willing to do a complete physical, including a variety of blood tests and a CT scan. She said we'd both be better able to cope if we knew what we were dealing with and could share our concerns with others.

She was right.

Local organized support or self-help groups are scattered all over the United States, wherever family members provide care. They meet in homes, hospitals, nursing homes, and churches. They come in all shapes and sizes, adapting themselves to the various needs represented by group members. Some are formal, with highly structured programs. Others are informal discussions. Some are a combination of the two.

Regardless of their structure, support groups are made up of other people who can prop you up when you are weary. When I called the local support group, I discovered that Dad and I weren't alone. There were many other people in the county, some even in our own neighborhood, who really understood our situation. They were *in* our situation.

Sometimes you feel like you're the only person in the world with a family situation like yours. And then you go to a support-group meeting and you realize there are other people very much like you.

Sometimes I get very lonely. I have friends, but they're not the same as the friends I've made through the support group. I find I need both.

Support groups can contribute to our own emotional and spiritual well-being.

After a while you begin to wonder if you're seeing things in the proper perspective. You feel like you're dealing with something all by yourself. But when you're able to talk with other people and listen to their experiences, you realize you're still okay yourself. You're not going off the deep end.

The support group was a place where I could share my real feelings. Even the negative ones—my guilt and my pain. No one ever said, "You shouldn't feel that way," because they all knew exactly what I was feeling. And why.

Support groups can offer us more than just a listening ear. Often their help comes in very practical, material ways.

The generosity of the support group overwhelmed me. They raised the money for our travel and the overnight stay in a motel when I had to take my husband to a research center to be involved in an experimental drug trial.

We laugh a lot in our support group. Not at our loved ones, but at some of the things they do. Many things are funny, though usually not at the time, when we're usually angry and frustrated. But after it's all over we need to be able to share. And to laugh. You can't do that with everyone. Some people would get offended and would think we have some sick sense of humor. But most of us realize laughter is therapy.

Support groups can even help with difficult decisions, such as whether to institutionalize our loved one or request a brain autopsy.

The support group guided me to a special psychiatric hospital where my husband is now. One support-group member, who knew I couldn't face the fact that my husband needed institutionalization, said to me, "Have you considered the psychiatric hospital? My wife has been there for ten years and she has received excellent care. Don't let preconceptions about 'mental institutions' prevent you from looking into it."

I called that hospital. I never would have done that without encouragement. It's a great place.

Through the support group I first heard about the need for brain autopsies and how to make arrangements. The group helped me sort through my feelings and make a decision.

Support groups are not only for caregivers whose loved ones are still living. Many groups include surviving spouses and relatives. Their reasons for continued involvement are varied.

My wife died four years ago and I still go to the support group. I feel that, having gone through all this, maybe I can help someone else. I think that's the way we all feel who have lost spouses or parents. Our trials are over, but maybe we can help someone whose trials aren't.

The support group fulfills a need in me to help other people. I hope that the little I can share can help relieve the problems of others.

Support groups aren't just for people who care for loved ones at home. Many caregivers whose loved ones are in nursing homes or adult homes continue to attend meetings.

> There are a lot of people who come to our support group who have relatives in nursing homes. Sometimes visiting loved ones in a nursing home is harder than if they were home with you. It's a different kind of hard. We still need support.

> The group I belong to actually meets in the nursing home where my mother is staying. It's great. The social worker leads it and we have the opportunity to ask questions. They bring in different speakers and we learn a lot.

Support groups aren't something you should feel obligated to join. There may be a wrong time or a right time to take part.

> My first experience at a support-group meeting was traumatic. I didn't want to hear about what might happen to my husband. He wasn't that bad yet, and I couldn't face the thought that he might be tied to a chair all day, playing with his shoelaces. He was still driving at the time and I didn't want to hear how bad it was going to be. I went to the group once and then came back, a year later. Then I was ready to hear.

> I'm a very private person. I just can't share my feelings in a group. I went once and felt uncomfortable. But I do keep in touch with several of the support-group members. That helps a lot.

Groups can be helpful even if you don't think you'd be comfortable voicing your concerns in front of others, or if you simply can't get out because of caregiving responsibilities.

> I wasn't able to get out to the support group for two years; I didn't have anyone to care for my wife. So the group came individually and visited me. I will always be grateful.

As the foregoing caregivers have mentioned, most support groups have members who are willing to talk on the telephone, send information, or channel you to appropriate resources and literature. They can also offer suggestions on management issues and other caregiver concerns, like finances and nursing home placement. And sometimes group members do make home visits to encourage caregivers who cannot come to meetings.

Support groups aren't just for adults. They can also include teenagers. If there are a number of caregivers with teens, consider establishing a separate group for the young people. If guidance is needed, it might be available through a group member or someone else in the community, such as a pastor or a psychologist. Bringing teens and parents together for an informal picnic or potluck might be a good place to start. *Alzheimer's Disease, Especially for Teenagers* is a brochure available from the Alzheimer's Association. (See appendix A for other helpful references if you have younger children or teens in your family.)

Last, support groups can help you feel more in control of what seems to be an uncontrollable situation. They can help you get actively engaged in the battle against Alzheimer's in a variety of ways.

> Our local group does a lot in the community. We sponsor workshops, supply speakers for churches and service clubs, distribute literature at health fairs and even our county fair. We help educate the community and increase awareness.

> Through the support group I learned how to be more involved politically, and how I could take my experience of pain and make a small difference in the world. I've written letters to congressmen about the financial needs of Alzheimer's families.

Then I went to some state hearings. One of these days I might even have the courage to testify.

The motto of the national Alzheimer's Association is "Someone to stand by you." The motto for local support groups could well be "Someone to walk with you." That is what Alzheimer's support groups have to offer.

Friends and Relations

Some caregivers report that their circle of friends has become more restricted as a result of their loved ones' illness. Others have discovered many new friendships. One thing is certain for all: if it weren't for friends to confide in, caregiving would be a very lonely business.

> I have a wonderful friend I can go to at any time. It started three years ago when she fell and broke her hip. After she came home from the hospital, I went every day and helped her put on her shoes and stockings. Sometimes I'd go early in the morning before my husband got out of bed. Other times I'd take him with me. I'd wash her feet, maybe cut her toenails, and we'd talk. She told me once, "I want to pay you for helping me." And I said to her, "Are you crazy? Don't you know how much a good psychiatrist costs? I should be paying you!" She is wonderful. She simply listens.

Neighbors and relatives can also be helpful when we need a short break in the day's care.

> I had a neighbor who was very good to us. I'd take my wife over once a week and she'd just sit and watch TV. She was no trouble at all, the neighbor said. No trouble at all.

> Our neighbor always had an open door, which was good because my mother wandered through it a lot! The neighbor sat

her down, got her a cup of coffee, and called us to say my mother was there and all right.

My daughter-in-law's a hairdresser. Every Saturday she does my wife's hair at her house, which is not the easiest thing to do, because my wife gets up about five or six times and wanders around. That's my vacation time. It's the only chance I get during the week to mow the lawn or to talk on the phone without getting interrupted.

Sometimes friends and neighbors might avoid us. Often this happens because of their own emotional response to Alzheimer's disease, not because of an uncaring attitude or rudeness. Visits with a person with Alzheimer's may remind our friends and neighbors of their own advancing age and mortality, two things many people would like to forget. Reasons for what caregivers perceive to be fair-weather friends or neglectful neighbors vary.

I really wanted to visit, but I didn't do it very much. I know my best friend's wife thought it was a lack of caring on my part. It wasn't. I was just plain scared. Now that he's dead I feel guilty. What can I say?

The same may be true of relatives who you may feel have abandoned your sinking ship and are shirking their responsibility. Caregivers often express feelings of anger, resentment, and frustration because of perceived abandonment. However, relatives may simply be unable to face their own fears and their loved one's failing health and frailty.

You should have seen my wife's brother. He was hotter than blazes when he found out she was in a nursing home. When he finally went up and saw her, she didn't know him. He said to me, "I didn't know she was this bad." I said, "I've been trying to tell you for three years, but you wouldn't believe me." Later he told me he didn't *want* to believe it.

It bothers me that my oldest child hasn't been to see his grandmother in over three years. But he can't seem to take it. He gets emotional when he's there and he starts to cry. And he's thirty-eight years old. On one hand, I think he should make himself go. But then, I suppose, she doesn't know him anyway. Maybe it doesn't matter.

In our case it's been much harder for the two oldest siblings to visit. They can't face it. In a dire emergency they might be of help, but not now, not on a steady basis. They're dealing with their own concerns about their future and also their own hurt and pain in facing the current situation. I know it's very painful. I hurt too. It's especially hard on my father and mother.

My brother lives in another state and, when he calls, he never talks about Dad. He keeps it inside.

One day he did visit, and he went with us to the nursing home. He didn't want to go, but I said to him, "You've been away for several years and you have no idea what's going on. I think it would be a good idea if you went out to see Dad. In fact, maybe you think it's a lot more gruesome than it actually is."

So my brother went with us and we sat and talked to Dad, or, rather, my mother and I sat and talked to Dad. I don't think my brother could understand how we could be so cool about it. We talked and laughed and fed Dad lunch while the kids were in the background, banging on the piano. My brother sat and watched us and didn't say a word. At one point I said, "Are you glad you came?" and he said, "Yes," and that was the end of that.

It's sad because I think my brother has been dying inside all these years. His best friend says he won't talk about it to him either. Maybe he's handling it. I hope so.

We'd all like to think that a chronic illness such as Alzheimer's would bring families and friends closer together, not pull them apart. It can do both, depending to some extent on our attitudes as caregivers and our willingness to understand and help our other loved ones. We may, at times, have to be gentle and forgiving in the midst of our own emotional upheavals. Life is too short and relationships are too valuable to carry grudges.

Yet sometimes the problem isn't difficulty dealing with emotions at all. Not everyone is comfortable being a caregiver or being around people who are physically or mentally impaired. Families and friends may not know what they can do. They may feel awkward. Or they may want to help but fear they'll be invading our privacy. Sometimes they need us to give them permission to help us. We can do this by asking them for assistance or advice.

There are many ways friends and relations can offer support to their loved one and to the primary caregiver. One caregiver told me how her whole family gets involved in their mother's care, even though they are separated by distance. Geography doesn't seem to be a barrier for this family. Though distance precludes day-to-day care, they make periodic visits and work together as a team.

One sibling is the problem solver. He uses his expertise to help with financial and legal problems. Another sibling is the organizer. She helped get her parents enrolled in a senior center and nutrition program, and she organized information about an experimental drug program her mother became involved with.

Another is the practical manager. She takes her mother shopping when she visits, alters clothing, and takes home special laundry, helping in practical ways.

A fourth sibling is the sounding board, the listener. She visits for a month at a time, offering encouragement and emotional support.

Sometimes this support springs up naturally and spontaneously. In other situations, it's good to have a family planning conference early in the disease process. This will help identify and coordinate the skills family members can contribute as the disease progresses and their loved one's needs increase.

Contributing to loved ones' financial needs is one way some relatives can share in the caregiving burden. Caregiving is expensive. Even if most of the bills are paid by some type of insurance or social-service program (an exception rather than a rule for most caregivers), there are always items that are not reimbursable, for example, adult briefs, special foods, and wheelchair repair.

Family members living in other parts of the country often attend support groups themselves. This gives them a more realistic picture of what the primary caregiver is coping with and what their loved one is suffering. In addition, they can learn more about Alzheimer's disease by attending conferences and exchanging audiotapes. Information they acquire can be shared across the miles.

Never underestimate the value of letters and phone calls. For the primary caregiver the feeling of aloneness doesn't lessen as the years go by—no matter how involved one may be in the community or in a support group. Tangible notes of support and encouragement help maintain and strengthen family ties.

Caregiving really is a family affair. It is a time for sharing, caring, and bearing each other's burdens in practical, tangible ways.

Little Ones

My five-year-old grandson loves his grandmother. When my daughter takes him to the nursing home to visit, he'll climb up on my wife's lap and kiss her. Then she'll smile, just like old times. He's the only one who can make her smile like that. He can be out in the hall and my wife will recognize his voice. She'll even yell at the nurses, "That's my boy. Let him come!" My wife always calms down when he comes.

I told my grandson that I wished we could have his grandmother back home again with us. You know what he said to me? He said, "That's all right, Grandpa. Grandma's sick. But that don't stop me from loving her."

Newborns. Infants. Toddlers. School-age children. Teens. If you have any children in your family or can borrow some from your friends, they can be a source of joy for both you and your loved one. Relating to your loved one can likewise be a joy for them.

Occasionally, children will be frightened by their grandmother's or grandfather's bizarre behavior, but most of the time they'll take it in stride and accept it.

Mom and her four-year-old grandson get along just fine. To a four-year-old, everything is new in the world and everything is as it should be. Therefore, if Grandma is confused and forgetful, that's okay. It must be normal. We'll accept that behavior. And so he does.

When I hired some home-care aides for my mother a number of years ago, one of the workers had two children, ages seven and nine. She brought them to work in the summer, and they always came over after school during the school year. Mom called them "cute little fellers" (a phrase she also used when referring to the squirrels on our deck, and even some of my older friends). But they didn't seem to mind. She also patted them on the head a lot and gave them hugs. They accepted her terms of endearment and responded in kind. To them, she was "Gramma."

Once I got home from work and discovered Mom and the two children hard at work on a special project that the children themselves had instituted. They'd brought over their coloring books and had also bought one for my mom. The three of them were having a great time coloring at the kitchen table. My mother the artist was once again at work.

As the months went by, my mother lost her ability to hold on to crayons. While her coloring lasted, it was a joy to watch her interact with the children for even short periods of time and to see the children care about her, accepting some of Mom's other behaviors as a normal part of life for a "grandmother" with Alzheimer's.

A week before my father died, one of the children wrote my mother a letter. It seems a fitting reminder of the importance of children in the lives of our loved ones—a reminder of what love is all about:

Dear Pearl:

Hi How are you today. I love you a lot. You are my best Friend. You are more Than a Friend. you are Like a Grama to me and all way be a Grama to me. Because I Love you so much. you will allways Be in my Heart. you are so Loveable & soft and so warm. and you allways will be in my Heart and in my Dreams. an so Does God Love you Like I Do. He Love's you to. He Does me and He Will allway's Look over you if I can't. He will allways watch over you pearl because I love you. and I love God to.

From Tanya L. Rood to pearl

Note: To find out about support groups in your area, contact your area or county office on aging, your community health home nursing agency, or the area Alzheimer's Association. These organizations can help you start a support group if there are none in your area.

Chapter 11

Resources for Regrouping

Elaine remembered when she loved her job. When it had been, in fact, her respite. But lately the tensions at work were unbearable. There was always the constant backbiting and bickering. And there were the stupid, hateful things the other women said about their husbands.

If they only knew, Elaine thought bitterly. *They should be grateful they have husbands. They should come home with me. See what it's like to live with a husband who doesn't even know your name. They'd begin to appreciate what they've got in a hurry. I wonder if anyone would take me up on the offer if I did invite them home.*

Home. Thinking of home, Elaine wondered how the new home-care aide was making out. The previous one lasted only a week. She turned in her resignation to the agency the day Steven locked her out of the house. He had unlocked the kitchen door in the morning and run out into the back yard. When the aide ran after him, Steven ran back into the kitchen, slamming and locking the door.

The aide spent two hours pleading with Steven to let her in. But Steven just stood there, smiling and waving at her. When the aide saw him turn the gas on under an empty frying pan, she had the presence of mind to run to the neighbor's house and call the police. And then she called her agency.

Despite the problems, Elaine didn't know what she'd have done without the home-health agency. The aides had been so good to Steven. One of them even joked about losing ten pounds the first week she cared for him. It made Elaine feel guilty, until the aide reassured her it was the best thing to happen to her figure in years.

But people in their forties weren't supposed to need home-care aides. They weren't supposed to get Alzheimer's disease. Cancer maybe, or diabetes, or a heart attack. Terrible things, too, but all potentially treatable. Not Alzheimer's. Not this horrible disease that turned you into some kind of hyperactive child.

When had it first begun? When did she first notice the signs? It wasn't until Steven received the letter from the school board requesting his resignation that reality finally hit her.

The absent-minded professor, the kids called Steven at school. At first it showed in little things. He would correct their exams and forget to give them grades. Then he went through one semester without giving an exam at all. The students never told. The school board accidentally found out about Steven's memory lapses when one of the board members overheard his daughter talking to a friend about the strange and wonderful chemistry professor.

Finally the day came when, in the middle of chemistry lab, Steven threw a beaker at a student in a fit of frustration. Fortunately, the only thing in the beaker was water. It was supposed to have have been acid, but Steven had forgotten the formula.

Now Elaine could look back and see other changes. There were initially problems with words. Steven always seemed to be searching to find the noun or the phrase to end a sentence. It started to drive Elaine crazy. Half the time she didn't know what he was talking about. And there were personality changes. The frustration. The angry outbursts for no apparent reason.

She remembered the Saturday morning Steven went to the store for a quart of milk and returned six hours later. She had really lit into him, accusing him of everything under the sun. And Steven just looked at her, then went into the bedroom, slammed and locked the door and stayed there until after dark. That happened just before they got the letter from the school board.

Two years later, here they were. Alone in a world where nothing made sense anymore. Maybe she should have listened to her mother and had a child. But no. She and Steven had both felt that all they wanted was each other and their careers. They were planning to take a trip around the world in three more years. No strings. No children. Each other.

Elaine opened her desk and reached for her purse. Time to go home. Home to the man she still loved beyond distraction and who didn't even know her name.

Purse. Leftover lunch. Library book. Bible. *Yes, I really should take that Bible home with me and read it,* Elaine thought. Once that was all that kept her sane, kept her going. But lately she'd gotten out of the habit of reading. Still, Elaine carted the Bible to the office each day, thinking that maybe this lunch hour she would find some time. She certainly never found time at home.

Where was that passage? Ah, yes. Isaiah 54, verses five and eight. "Your Creator will be like a husband to you—the Lord Almighty is his name. The holy God of Israel will save you. . . . 'I will show you my love for ever.' So says the Lord who saves you."

The Lord, her husband. Not Steven. Not anymore. At least not in the sense that he could meet her needs for friendship or companionship. Not Steven, her husband, but the Lord, her Maker.

As Elaine slipped the Bible into her purse, she fervently prayed that when she walked through her kitchen door in forty-five minutes, she would remember what the Lord had said to Israel—and have hope for her own life.

Short-Term Relief

You may think, as a number of caregivers have told me, that no one can care for your loved one as well as you can. This may be true. But if you are a parent you probably said the same thing when you hired your first baby sitter or sent your first child off to kindergarten. Much to your amazement, you both survived. You will survive this time too.

> Dad was very aggressive. He mellowed somewhat as he got older, but his temper got worse as the Alzheimer's disease came on. It was very hard on my mother. She was the type of person who would take everything and wouldn't fight back. But there were times when she would go into her room, shut the door, cry, and scream and scream—just to get rid of the tension. I don't know why she didn't have a nervous breakdown. Ten years, and no respite.

148

As Alzheimer's disease progresses, most caregivers will need some short-term relief as well as extended periods of respite. Friends or family members may be willing to fill in for long weekends. An extended getaway, however, requires more formal arrangements. A number of options are available to caregivers depending on where you live, your financial situation, and your needs.

All the available community services and service providers make it possible for us to keep our loved one at home for as long as it is safe and desirable. They are not designed to totally take away our caregiving responsibilities, but to give us the short-term help we need to rest, regroup, and recoup our personal strength and resources. We are then better equipped to manage at home when we return.

Home Care

Formal in-home services delivered through city, county, and community agencies include various types of nursing services, home-health and personal-care aides, respite workers, and homemakers/housekeepers. Mealtime help may be provided through Meals-on-Wheels or other nutrition programs that deliver hot and cold meals to people with disabilities.

Caregivers frequently cite the value of regularly scheduled home-care workers.

> Aides from a county home-care agency came in twice a week to give my husband a bath, shave him, and give him his breakfast. After breakfast, they'd take him for a walk. It was so good to have a couple hours to myself.

> I'm semi-retired and have a part-time teaching job two afternoons a week. I hired home-health aides from a private home-care agency when I finally realized I had to have someone with her when I was at work. My major support came from these home-health aides.

Home care was wonderful. It was my salvation. The girl that came was great. Fortunately, my husband was on Medicaid so we were able to have aide help eight hours a day, five days a week. And I worked outside the home every day.

My work was really my respite. I couldn't have stood being home all day long.

If you're looking for in-home services, the following tips may apply.

➤ Talk with other caregivers who have hired helpers. What services have they used? Were the services reliable and dependable?

➤ Call your county, community or public-health nursing service, office on aging, or department of social services. They can tell you what services are available through their agencies and whether they are reimbursable through federal, state, or county funding programs.

➤ Most county agencies also work closely with various community-aide agencies. If the people you call can't provide services directly, they should be able to refer you to agencies that can.

➤ If you need home-care help following the hospital discharge of your loved one, contact the hospital's discharge planner or social worker as soon as possible. This person can help you make post-hospital arrangements and is also a good agency referral source.

There are a number of advantages to hiring through an established, reputable agency. These include:

• registered nurse supervision of home-care workers
• development of an in-home plan of care to meet your specific needs
• formal training of home-care workers
• provision of substitute workers if the scheduled worker is ill
• payment of the workers' taxes, social security, and liability insurance

- payment of all or part of the home-care expenses if you fit the income eligibility and/or medical criteria, especially Medicaid
- provision of various levels of service ranging from cooking, cleaning, and shopping to direct personal caregiving

Turn the above advantages into questions for the agency when you ask about information and services.

In one of its informative brochures, the National Home Care Association raises additional questions that are good to ask when hiring through an agency:

1. How long has the agency served the community?
2. What is its reputation?
3. Is the agency certified by Medicare or licensed by the state health department? Certified and licensed agencies must meet certain minimum requirements for financial management and patient care and are monitored by the state on a regular basis.
4. Is written information available about the agency's services, eligibility requirements, fees, and funding sources?

The National Home Care Association can be contacted at 228 7th Street S.E., Washington, DC 20003, (202) 547-7424. They can help you contact your state home-care association, which will have information about certified and licensed agencies in your area.

Cutting the Costs

Agency home care can be paid for through a number of different sources. *Medicare* is a federal health-care program for people over the age of sixty-five. Your loved one must be under a physician's care, be homebound, and meet other eligibility criteria to qualify. In addition, services must be provided by Medicare-certified agencies.

Because of the custodial nature of the care given most Alzheimer's sufferers, Medicare generally won't pay unless your loved one has been recently hospitalized or suffers from some other, more acute condition. Some health insurance policies provide home-care coverage, though most, like Medicare, are geared for acute rather than chronic conditions.

If your loved one is a military veteran or the spouse of a veteran, check with the *Veterans Administration*. They have a number of medical benefits that include home care.

Most states also have a *medical-assistance program* for low-income people (for example, Medicaid or, in California, Medi-Cal). Every state has its own set of eligibility requirements. If your loved one is eligible, Medicaid provides some of the best home-care coverage around. Some people who have an income too high to qualify initially may be able to go through a "spend-down" process to become eligible. Don't eliminate this automatically until you've talked with your county social-service department.

Many home-care expenses are *tax deductible* for spouses and children who are primary caregivers. Contact the Internal Revenue Service. Be sure to save all medically related receipts and keep accurate records of expenses.

If agency help is not available or affordable, as is often the case, you can also *hire privately*. Many men and women with tender hearts and good skills are looking for home-care jobs. These people may have been trained through on-the-job experience with home-care agencies, or in hospitals or nursing homes.

Most newspapers have ads from home-care workers seeking independent employment. These workers may be trained or certified aides, though training itself is not necessarily an indication of how reliable or how honest an aide will be. Avoid hiring over the phone. It's best to have applicants come to your home for a personal preemployment interview. Are they able to physically manage your loved one? Find out about any health problems. Will they need to do heavy lifting? Can they? Discuss fees (they will usually set an hourly rate) based on what they want, what you can afford, and what you believe is the going rate in your area. If you hire privately you may be liable to pay state or federal taxes and Social Security. Check with a tax adviser, the IRS, and Social Security.

To minimize risks, ask prospective employees for several references, preferably previous employers, and call them. A good aide will not mind this or feel that it's an intrusion. Communicate with other caregivers who may have hired help in the past. A "caregivers' grapevine" can let you know who's reliable and who's not.

Nursing schools or high-school prenursing programs can be good sources of home-care help. Students are often looking for part-time employment. Sometimes they are also looking for a place to live. For two years I had a student live with us. In exchange for room, board, and a negotiated salary, she cared for my mother, saved for a year of college, and enabled me to hold down a full-time job. She had weekends and evenings off but was always willing to help me out when I needed some extra time for myself.

Advertise for help in the newspaper. Place your name with the local nursing school, nursing home, or hospital. Hospitals and nursing homes sometimes hire aides who desire full-time employment on only a part-time basis; they may be looking for additional employment in the community.

Adult Day Care

"If only there had been a place where I could have left my mother for the day. I simply needed a day off now and then," said one caregiver. There *are* places to leave our loved ones for a day. Adult day-care programs provide socialization, a nutritious meal, and a structured and supervised environment with a wide range of activities.

Availability, criteria for eligibility, and the cost of day-care services vary widely from state to state and county to county, but they are usually a very economical—perhaps the *most* economical—form of help for the caregivers.

Some adult day-care centers are run by the local office on aging or community groups; others may be affiliated with and located in hospitals or nursing homes. Some centers care for all older people with physical and intellectual impairment. Others are only for those with physical disabilities or people with dementia. Payment for day care is usually private or through Medicaid.

One job I held necessitated a two-hour drive once a month for management meetings. The meeting was in Albany, our state capital. I inquired about day-care options and found a center, which catered exclusively to Alzheimer's sufferers, only a few blocks from our meeting place. So Mom went with me on the monthly trips. She loved the ride and seemed to thrive in the center's environment.

I loved it too: eight hours later I was only fifteen dollars poorer. Home care would have cost me four to five times as much for the twelve hours away from home. If you do any traveling, think about this option and call ahead to learn about available services.

Adult homes are another option. These are usually family-owned homes, regulated by county social service departments, that provide live-in, twenty-four-hour help for the frail elderly. Some exclusively take in people with Alzheimer's. Some are willing to care for people only during the day, on an occasional overnight, or for several weeks or a month of respite for needy caregivers. I used this option about twice a month at an affordable cost. Your social service department will have an official listing, though there may be homes which aren't officially licensed but which give excellent care. Once again, ask around.

Another option I discovered was the "sitter/companion." Some mothers who are home with their children don't mind another mouth to feed at lunch and, if your loved one is manageable and doesn't wander, would see him or her as a welcome addition to their home. I used this arrangement once a week and I paid her a regular rate. I dropped Mom off in the morning, went to work at the nursing home and returned around nine at night, taking some time for myself. Mom seemed to enjoy her times with the children, and they liked to be with her. My refrigerator was covered with "pictures for Pearle" that one little girl kept giving us. Ask around. Check references.

Other Alternatives

You may also want to consider some alternative options for the care of your loved one. Some hospitals, nursing homes, and adult homes provide respite care for caregivers on a short-term basis. Respite care is temporary, twenty-four-hour care that allows caregivers time for rest. If this service is not available in your area, your support group might consider it a worthy lobbying effort. It can be a wonderful relief for a caregiver who is ill or needs a real vacation.

An exchange-a-loved-one program with other caregivers in your support group may be possible. It may not be any more difficult or time-consuming to care for two or even three people with Alzheimer's than to care for one. In fact, there may be *less* care involved.

At the various day-care centers and adult homes I've used or visited, I've seen that people with Alzheimer's have a language all their own; they often communicate very well with each other, especially in the later stages of the disease. In fact, they may find it a relief to care for each other and talk to each other, and the caregivers' burden is lessened.

Some caregivers have tried a number of the foregoing options and have had negative experiences. This is to be expected. We know that caring for someone with Alzheimer's is not easy. Not everyone can do it. Even some trained personnel may never have encountered dementia.

We needn't let one or even several rough experiences sour us to all substitute caregivers. Sooner or later we'll wind up with the perfect match and probably wonder how we ever managed without the support of that particular home-care agency, home-health aide, or day-care program.

That's as it should be as we shift the caregiving responsibility onto someone else's shoulders for a while and take a needed break.

God, the Ultimate Resource

I heard a story once about a nurse who was caring for children. One little boy, confined to an oxygen tent, was not only having difficulty breathing, he was terrified by the whole experience of confinement.

The nurse had a solution. She opened the tent flaps and crawled in beside the screaming toddler. Sensing her presence, the comfort of another human being, the child promptly fell asleep.

As caregivers, we may feel a lot like that screaming little boy. We may not have difficulty breathing, but we do have difficulty coping with the day-to-day responsibilities that threaten to overwhelm us. We feel claustrophobic, confined, and terrified. We desperately long for someone to "climb into our tent with us" and give us comfort or, better yet, set us free.

Sometimes we can escape from our emotionally charged tent for a few hours. We may get out of the house, shop, golf, dine with friends, or attend a support-group meeting. But unfortunately not all of us can get out. Even if we do, we still need support and understanding when the door closes behind us back home—where we're alone with our loved ones.

Our freedom is illusory. But there is a resource, one we might think of as our ultimate support system. That ultimate resource is God.

Various polls indicate that over ninety percent of Americans believe in God. What the polls don't indicate is what kind of God the American people believe in. Beliefs are diverse.

For some, God is a cosmic watchmaker who has made the universe, wound it up, then left it to tick along on its own. This God is no longer involved with the world he has created.

Others view God as a vague, impersonal energy force who didn't *create* the universe, but who *is* the universe. In other words, there is really no difference between God, a person, a turtle, or a turnip—all creation is One. God is everything and everything is God.

A third view, if in fact it can be called a view of God at all, is that there is no God. Human beings, according to this view, are on the highest rung of the evolutionary ladder. Faith in God has been replaced by faith in people, who are thought to be the measure of all things.

These are three very different views of God, but they have one thing in common. None offers hope to the caregiver who is struggling to make sense out of suffering, and who needs support and encouragement in the struggle.

The Bible's picture of God is different. God can be a source of hope. The Bible claims that God cares personally about us. He is the Creator of the universe and distinct from it. He is nevertheless actively involved in the universe. All creation is under his control.

I really don't know how people can function without God in their lives. I overheard someone mention that Jesus was just a crutch people used. I thought, *so what's wrong with that?* If you're crippled, you need something to lean on. And I'm crippled. I think we all are.

I don't think anything in life would make sense without believing in Jesus Christ. I think of my father. You live your life, you're alert, you give to society, and then all of a sudden your body and mind start giving way. My father's illness wouldn't make sense without God. Without God there would be no justice.

I do a fair amount of Bible reading. I love it. And I keep finding little notes to myself I've jotted down as reminders of who God is to me. He's my refuge, one note says. He's my strength. God is my salvation.

If I hadn't had a relationship with God—a *personal* relationship—I couldn't have gone on.

The God these caregivers are talking about has something in common with that nurse who comforted the little boy in the oxygen tent by going in beside him. Nearly two thousand years ago, God came beside his people in the person of Jesus Christ. Jesus became a human being who came into our hurting world and experienced pain and suffering as we have. Why did God do that? There are several reasons.

God wanted to show us what he is like. It's pretty difficult to relate to an invisible God, even though evidence of his character is all around us. Jesus solved that problem by being God visible, God as a human being. By reading the four accounts of Jesus by Matthew, Mark, Luke and John in the New Testament, we can get an accurate picture of what God is really like. We learn, through Jesus, that God is loving, perfect, and just. He's a Father who cares about his children, who is beside them in their suffering and comforts their fears.

God came to meet our deepest needs as human beings. Regardless of what our popular culture tells us, we are not God. That means we are not sufficient unto ourselves. We all have the need to make sense of life in general and of suffering in particular; the need for love and relationship; the need for safety and security; the need for hope in the present and for the future; and the need to be free from guilt, resentments, depression, fears, and anxieties.

We often look to other people to meet these needs for us. But ultimately people fail us. They can ignore us, desert us, get sick, or die. Other people often create in us the very needs we turn to them to meet! It all boils down to one simple fact: Jesus alone is the only one who can meet our deepest needs, the needs that really matter.

God came to bring eternal life. This life filled with pain and suffering is not the end of things. There's another life to come—one in which God has promised to wipe every tear from our eyes—in a place where there will be no more death, no more mourning, no more crying, no more pain. (Revelation 21:4). And, we can assume, no more Alzheimer's disease.

One caregiver I interviewed told me of her experience.

> I joined a small group to strengthen my own faith, and I found it was like going to a well once a week and getting replenished. I love that metaphor of getting fresh water for my soul, refreshing myself as I learn about God with others.
>
> I'm finding things in the Bible that mean different things, now that my husband has Alzheimer's. I can personalize the things I'm reading. I can apply the teachings of Jesus to my life.
>
> Right now I'm reading in the book of Isaiah. It has taken me two weeks just to go through one chapter. I find myself reading it over and over, like I'm digging deeper and deeper into a really deep well. As I read, I find more and more riches.
>
> I can't get to the small group much anymore because I need to be home for my husband. I miss the give-and-take discussion and learning together. But I know that I can always go to God on my own.

The image of a well that refreshes and replenishes is a fitting metaphor for a relationship with Jesus. "Whoever is thirsty," Jesus said, "should come to me and drink. . . . Whoever believes in me, streams of lifegiving water will pour out from his heart." (John 7:37-39, TEV). This kind of relationship with Jesus can be an ultimate source of hope.

We may need to be reminded at times that God truly does love us and our loved ones. He cares about our confusion and the emotional pain we have as caregivers. He wants to carry us through it.

Chapter 12

Our Tangled Emotions

I remember sitting in the kitchen with my two-year-old, feeling miserable, when a song about a woman who had died started playing on the radio. I started sobbing.

My emotions were all bottled up inside. That song triggered them. I went outside, sat on the steps for half an hour and cried and cried. I couldn't stop. There was all this pent-up emotion. I knew it was because of my mother.

Our emotional responses to Alzheimer's are often as mixed up and tangled as the minds of our loved ones. Sometimes we need help to sort through them and straighten them out.

Fear. Anxiety. Guilt. Anger. Depression. These are the primary emotions caregivers experience. But the full picture needn't look so bleak. What we may perceive as negative emotions are a natural, if uncomfortable, response to our loss of a loved one. What we are doing, in fact, is *grieving*. And grief is healthy and normal.

Granger Westberg, in his popular book *Good Grief*, wrote about the emotions people feel when facing the loss of a loved one. He noted that there are good and bad ways to grieve, healthy and unhealthy emotions to experience. Grief is a "road the majority of humans must travel in order to get back into the mainstream of life."[1] That applies to caregivers.

To be free from worry and anxiety in the face of uncertainty, to be at peace with our loved ones without feeling resentful or resigned—these are healthy signs that we have come to terms with our conflicting emotions. They show that we are truly experiencing "good" grief.

Fears and Anxieties

Fear and anxiety are common emotional reactions when a loved one is diagnosed with Alzheimer's. They are strongest among children of Alzheimer's sufferers.

The question *"Is Alzheimer's disease hereditary?"* is asked by every son and daughter. We pray the answer is no. We fear the answer is yes. Fear and anxiety may increase if we know our family history.

> I think it may be the fourth generation for my mother. Her mother died when she was sixteen. We're sure it was Alzheimer's. My mother's grandmother had the same symptoms. Judging from the family anecdotes we've been gathering, a great-uncle had symptoms too.

The fear becomes even greater if we, too, become forgetful.

> Sometimes I forget the names of people I should know, and that terrifies me. My wife sees the look that comes over my face and she says, "Now, don't start getting upset."

Many caregivers can cope by joking about the possibility of Alzheimer's. Others use their knowledge to plan for the future.

> My two sisters and I crack jokes about how we'll be the old Alzheimer's gals. We'll get a home together.

> I'm not really afraid of getting Alzheimer's. If I do, I hope I have enough lucid moments in the beginning so that I'll have time to make plans and take care of everything. I certainly don't sit around and worry. I do, occasionally, think about planning for the future.

I kid about it with my roommate sometimes. She'll say to me, "You're acting funny again. Sign the paper." We make a joke of it.

I did tell her that, if I ever start acting as my father did, I want to sign the paper so someone will have power of attorney over me.

Sometimes the more we know about the disease, the less we're able to cope with it. Other people can help put our fears and anxieties in perspective.

I read some information about Alzheimer's disease that said I had a good chance of getting Alzheimer's because my mother had it. Then I went to a conference where they talked about the heredity factor. I was so depressed when I came home, I spent the next four days in bed.

A friend said, "Are you going to make your husband and your children miserable for the next twenty years just because you think you might get it? You'll ruin your lives. And besides, you could get hit by a bus tomorrow. A plane could fall from the sky. You simply can't worry about getting this disease."

Are fear and anxiety justified? Is Alzheimer's hereditary? What are the risks to children of Alzheimer's sufferers and to future generations?

Studies have demonstrated an increased risk of developing Alzheimer's among those who have Alzheimer's in their family. Those closest to the person with Alzheimer's are at a slightly higher risk than relatives several generations removed. According to one study, the overall risk of acquiring Alzheimer's disease is about four times greater if you have a first-degree relative (parents, siblings, children) with dementia. Although this risk to even first-degree relatives is still very small, it increases as people reach their seventies and eighties. Some relatives of Alzheimer's sufferers do develop dementias in later life. Others do not.[2]

Researchers are constantly looking for links between Alzheimer's and similar diseases. One area of genetic exploration is related to Down syndrome (previously "Down's syndrome") or mongolism, a hereditary condition accompanied by an extra chromosome that causes profound mental retardation.

The possible genetic thread linking both Alzheimer's disease and Down syndrome is the presence of a large number of senile plaques and neurofibrillary tangles present in brain tissue of both Alzheimer's and Down syndrome sufferers.

Autopsies on Down syndrome sufferers over the age of forty show evidence of the characteristic plaques and tangles of Alzheimer's disease—even if they didn't exhibit Alzheimer's when they were alive. This finding has sparked considerable interest and activity in genetic research that may one day uncover a cause and a cure for Alzheimer's.[3]

Rather than fear the genetic implications, we should welcome scientific advances and encourage the research that may help subsequent generations.

When his anxious and troubled followers worried about having their basic needs met, Jesus reminded them that God provides (Matthew 6:25-33). And if God provides rain for the earth and food for the animals, he can and will provide for us. He can give us the strength to be caregivers today and to face the future with peace.

The Guilt Trip

Psychiatrist Karl Menninger wrote about a man who stood on a busy street corner and repeated one word aloud, over and over again. The word was *guilty*. Each time the man said "Guilty," he'd point at a passerby. The accused people hesitated, looked away, then glanced furtively at each other—as if they actually felt guilty.[4]

Caregivers may feel a lot like those poor pedestrians. Whatever we say, wherever we go, whatever we do, we can't escape the pointing finger. If we don't think others are pointing it at us, we point it at ourselves. It's a no-win situation.

What makes us feel guilty? Dozens of things.

We feel guilty about our attitude toward our loved one's confusion, agitation, and behaviors.

I felt guilty every minute of the day. Not so much for the way I treated my mother, but for the things I thought about her. I didn't holler or scream, but I certainly felt like it at times. Her agitation, and especially the repetitiveness, drove me nuts.

I usually coped by walking out of the room, leaving my mother in her chair to talk to herself. I suppose you might call that neglect, but it was the only way I could handle my emotions.

I was never outright mean to my wife. I didn't physically abuse her. But I acted as if she didn't exist. She'd ask me a question for the twenty-fifth time in one morning and I'd just walk away. Ignoring her became a habit.

I felt guilty about it, a nagging, clawing kind of guilt.

Our behavior can bother us when we finally vent our pent-up emotions and verbally or even physically lash out at our loved ones in a caregiver's version of a catastrophic reaction.

I would be so very mean to my husband. I'd say cutting, hurtful things to him. I couldn't seem to stop myself. I was so frustrated.

I would get mad at my wife and feel badly later. I don't think you can help that. You're driven to extremes, then afterward you're sorry.

One time my wife bit me so hard I turned around and bit her on the shoulder. She had so many clothes on it didn't hurt her at all. It was just a sudden reaction on my part. Then I felt guilty.

The decision to place a loved one in a nursing home is often fraught with guilt, compounded by the promises we may have made to "never, ever do such a thing."

I think the hardest thing for me was taking my husband to the nursing home. He was still lucid enough to realize we were taking him away from his home, and he said, "I worked so hard all my life. Why are you doing this to me?" You can imagine how I felt, how I still feel.

Father used to say, "Don't ever put me in a nursing home. Take me out in the field and shoot me before you put me in one of those places."

So we told him we'd never do it. And then, one day, we did it.

I've read that people have taken care of their loved ones at home for seventeen years. So I felt guilty for not keeping him home. I still feel guilty whenever I visit him, especially if he's alert. But what could I do? I'm eighty-nine years old.

Wishing a parent, spouse, sister, or brother dead and out of their misery is not an uncommon source of guilt.

When my brother was still driving, I thought that maybe he'd drive off the cliff at the back of our house and it would be over for him. It would end his suffering. I never told anyone I had those thoughts.

Once my father was lost and my brother found him wandering down by the river. When he came home, my brother said to me, "I had the most horrible thoughts when we were searching. I hoped that Dad might have fallen in the river and that it was all over for him. I felt so guilty for thinking that way."

Neglected responsibilities make us feel guilty—floors to mop, the lawn to mow, letters to answer, and the bills to pay.

> I know my house is a wreck and I've let things pile up. Sometimes I get overwhelmed by depression. Most of the time I just feel guilty because I think I should be able to get my act together and keep things in order: my father, my house, my life.

> Our neighbors must think they live next to an abandoned building. Yard work is at the bottom of my priority list, and I feel ashamed of the way my house looks. Inside as well as outside.

Unmet family obligations and needs can create guilt for us.

> My husband was a brick through it all. Sometimes I wonder why he didn't ask for a divorce. I certainly didn't meet many of his needs for a whole year after my mother moved in with us. *Any* of his needs, if you know what I mean.

> It was hard on the children to grow up in the same house with a grandparent who had Alzheimer's. They never complained, but I know it was hard.
>
> We couldn't do anything together as a family, because someone had to stay home and watch Dad. I don't think I have any pictures from a family vacation. Vacations never happened. I feel bad about that.

Psychologists may tell us this caregiver guilt is false, related to the unrealistic expectations we have of ourselves. This may be true. But simply *calling* it false guilt doesn't help. And sorting false guilt from real guilt, when we're overwhelmed by both, can seem impossible.

At home we tried every day to give Dad a bath or just wash him up, but he'd always fight. When we took Dad to the nursing home, he had dirt in the creases of his neck. I was embarrassed.

When I visited him and looked at his neck, it was clean. I said, "Thank God," but I was embarrassed again!

Sometimes we need other people to help us sort through our guilt. A friend, members of our support group, counselors, and clergy can all be valuable sounding boards.

Yet when we're all talked out, supported, analyzed, and back home again, we may find that things really haven't changed. Our guilt hasn't walked away. We still respond the same way to the same situations. Guilt continues to incapacitate us emotionally and physically. It threatens to eat up our energy, buffet our bodies, and force us into self-condemnation and depression.

Good News

Guilt, even false guilt, is never benign. And, unfortunately, false guilt can be a smoke screen. It can effectively hide a deeper, underlying problem we have apart from our caregiving experiences. That problem is *true guilt*.

True guilt is not the result of things we do or don't do. True guilt is related to who we are. It is based on the fact that all of us have broken God's laws. We are all guilty of rebelling. We are like sheep that have wandered away from the shepherd.

The good news is that there's a cure for this disease of wandering from God—this *sin*—and its consequences. We can get rid of it by asking for God's forgiveness.

One of the most touching illustrations of what it means to have our sin and guilt washed away is told by Jeff Smith, host of the popular television program *The Frugal Gourmet*; Smith is also an ordained minister who often adds wisdom from theology to his cookbooks. He draws the following story from the ancient sheepherding communities of the Middle East.

During the night, mother ewes sometimes died giving birth to their lambs. At the same time, other mother ewes gave birth to still-born lambs. In the morning, a shepherd might find a newborn lamb languishing from lack of milk, while in another part of his flock he might find a grieving mother ewe.

"All logic would tell you," writes Smith, "to put the orphan under the care of the childless mother, . . . but the two would know they were foreign and would not accept each other."

A good shepherd solved this problem by draining the dead lamb's blood and washing the living orphan in it. Smelling the blood of her own offspring, the mother ewe would allow the orphan to suckle. She truly became the lamb's mother, and the orphan became her adopted child.[5]

This is a fascinating and beautiful illustration of what it means to have our sins forgiven and our guilt washed away, and to be adopted by God. As human beings we're separated from God by our sin. We're unable to rescue ourselves. We need someone to save us. For that reason, Jesus, God's son, was born to shed his blood for us when he died on the cross.

How can we take advantage of this sacrifice? We start by admitting that we can't save ourselves. We also have to believe that Jesus died to save us. In fact, Jesus conquered death on our behalf. He rose from the dead and he lives today, able to change our lives and shape our attitudes and behaviors. We need only ask.

People in every generation have asked God's forgiveness. Their prayers might help us voice our own responses to God.

> I look to the Lord for help at all times, and he rescues me from danger. Turn to me, Lord, and be merciful to me, because I am lonely and weak. Relieve me of my worries and save me from all my troubles. Consider my distress and suffering and forgive all my sins. (Psalm 25:15-18, TEV)

> From the depths of my despair I call to you, Lord. Hear my cry, O Lord; Listen to my call for help! If you kept a record of

our sins, who could escape being condemned? But you forgive us. (Psalm 131:1-4, TEV)

God, have mercy on me, a sinner. (Luke 18:13)

A modern-day caregiver describes her experience like this:

> I knew in my heart I was guilty. I knew I couldn't earn my way to God. So one night I just asked Jesus to forgive me and accept me. I felt real peace, a knowledge that what I had done was right.

Once we ask for forgiveness, we can be assured that God is in control of our lives and will strengthen us to weather any crisis. Without knowledge of God's love and support, we're left to "go it alone"— denying our guilt, rationalizing it, or dealing with it superficially. We're unable to draw on the forgiveness and strength that are ours as children of a gracious God.

The freedom that comes from being forgiven is more than simply not feeling guilty. It is the experience of new life and the promise of life to come. It is the realization that it's possible to have joy in the midst of mourning, hope in the midst of despair. It is knowing that the experience of caregiving does not have to devastate us. That is indeed good news.

Chapter 13

Hot But Not Burned Up

Over ten years ago I was working in a nursing home in Illinois as a spiritual-care coordinator. I loved my job, I loved the area, and I was in love. The fact that he wasn't equally in love with me was something I figured would work itself out in time. I was really looking forward to my future.

Then came the phone call.

"Sharon," said my aunt, my father's youngest sister, "you know you've always said to let you know if there were any problems on the home front. Well, there are. With your mother. I think it's time you moved back home." That was not news I wanted to hear.

I knew for years that my mother was having "a bit of a memory problem." I attributed it to her retirement, failing eyesight, and my dad's sudden onset of adult diabetes, an event that seemed to throw my mother into a state of confusion and anxiety. Alzheimer's disease was the furthest thing from my mind. I couldn't even spell it.

I received a lot of advice from friends and colleagues in Illinois. Even the administrator of the nursing home called me into her office. She gave me a very comforting lecture on how I needed to think about my needs, my future, my job.

"Perhaps you should call your father and talk to him about the possibility of nursing-home placement," she suggested. Take a short leave of absence, get things squared away at home, then come back to Illinois. Neat. Simple. Just what I wanted to hear.

That was not, however, what I was supposed to do. God, it seemed, had other plans for my life. He made them clear in no uncertain terms one night when I was reading the Bible.

In the book of Mark, Jesus was speaking to the religious leaders of the day. He was talking to them about their responsibility to their parents, and he called them hypocrites. They apparently gave money for temple offerings while their parents went hungry. They were, Jesus said, worshiping God in vain (Mark 7:1-13).

I felt convicted and doomed. I packed my bags—not eagerly, not happily—and drove home.

For the next several years I helped my father care for my mother. I either lived at home or shuffled back and forth between my parents' home and an apartment in a nearby city where I found a nursing job. Life seemed an unending merry-go-round of work, work, and more work as Mom's symptoms got worse, my father developed cancer, and I had to face the facts that I was probably back home for good, constantly caregiving and still very much single.

I was also very angry with God.

My primary support system had always been my church. I stopped going. The Bible had always been my point of strength. I stopped reading. Prayer had always been my source of encouragement. I stopped praying.

It was easy to justify my lack of church involvement. I had my parents as an excuse.

Justifying my lack of an ongoing relationship with God was harder. It was something I tried not to think about very much; I hoped no one would ask me about it. Few did. For months I continued being both angry and miserable. Then I finally came to terms with my feelings and began dealing with them constructively.

God isn't always the target of our anger. Sometimes we're angry at Alzheimer's itself, a disease we barely understand and cannot control.

I was angry at this disease that was destroying my father's mind. I was angry because life wasn't turning out the way I'd envisioned for my parents.

I quit smoking so I wouldn't get lung cancer. I changed my diet so I wouldn't have a heart attack. And here comes this disease that I have absolutely no control over. I can't do anything to prevent it. I realize no matter how healthy my lifestyle is, I won't be able to stop it or do anything about it if I get it. And because my mother has it, I look at myself as being a sitting duck.

It angers me. I know anger isn't going to do me any good, but it makes me so mad.

Sometimes our anger is directed at our loved ones, then at ourselves because we don't feel good about our angry outbursts. We want to change, but we struggle.

We were angry with my mother for the things she said and did. It would be so frustrating. She would ask the same questions over and over again until my father thought he'd go out of his mind. What day is it? What day is it? What month is it? What month is it? The same questions over and over.

Dad would say, "For Pete's sake, I told you the answer to that ten times already." Then he'd go into the bedroom and slam the door.

There's always a tendency, especially if there are other people around, to let your best side show, though inside you know things are different. I didn't want my patience to be a mask I was putting on.

When I got those feelings of anger and impatience, I didn't like it. Daddy knew he was irritating me. He'd try to apologize for something that wasn't his fault. I got very upset with myself for being angry and impatient with him when he'd ask me the same thing for the hundredth time.

When I got that way, I'd go into the bedroom and talk to God. I'd say, "Help me to be patient. Help me to remember. Help me to show Daddy the patience I'd want someone to show me."

Primary caregivers may feel they are the only ones who really care about their loved ones. Anger at other members of the family who "never call, never visit, never show any concern," is common.

I don't understand why my wife's brother never visits. For ten years she's had Alzheimer's. For five years she's been in the nursing home. He's never visited her there once. Not once.

In hospitals and nursing homes, anger is sometimes directed at health-care staff, doctors, nurses, or nursing assistants.

I got furious at some of the things the nurse's aides would say or do. You can't treat people like cattle, but that's the way they behaved at times. Especially at mealtimes. I'd see a few of them shoveling the food into patients' mouths and hear them say things like, "If you don't eat this they're going to send you to the hospital and put a tube down your nose."

Sometimes we even vent our frustrations on the furniture.

I never told my husband this, but the reason the mirror is broken in the bathroom is because I slammed the bathroom door so hard the mirror broke. I told him I was trying to kill a wasp with a broom handle. I think he believed me. I was just so ashamed of myself for getting so angry that I'd actually started destroying the furniture.

Not all expressions of anger are healthy. Our angry outbursts can hurt other people. They can also make us feel guilty and ashamed of ourselves. But the emotion of anger itself is not always unhealthy or destructive. Anger can be a legitimate response to justifiable causes.

What makes us angry? Why? These are the two key questions.

Anger at God

"Whenever there is suffering, whether physical pain or mental anguish, man-at-his-best will do his best to help. But his powers are so limited. God's power, so they say, is unlimited. So why doesn't He do something?" wrote Hugh Silvester in *Arguing with God*.[1]

C.S. Lewis, in his book *A Grief Observed*, also asked *why* when his wife was diagnosed with a fatal illness:

> What chokes every prayer and every hope is the memory of all the prayers (she) and I offered and all the false hopes we had. Not hopes raised merely by our own wishful thinking; hopes encouraged, even forced upon us, by false diagnoses, by x-ray photographs, by strange remissions, by one temporary recovery that might have ranked as a miracle. Step by step we were "led up the garden path."[2]

A bit earlier (three to four thousand years earlier), a man named Job also asked the *why* question as he sat on an ash heap, stricken by boils, grieving about his own physical suffering and the deaths of his ten children. He bitterly cried out against the apparent injustice of God:

> I am tired of living. Listen to my bitter complaint.
> Don't condemn me, God. Tell me!
> What is the charge against me?
> Is it right for you to be so cruel?
> To despise what you yourself have made?
> And then to smile on the schemes of wicked men?
> (Job 10:1-3, TEV)

Today, people with Alzheimer's, and their caregivers, are still asking, "Why?"

> My wife can't understand why everything happened to her the way it did. She said that if you believe in God, then things

should be nice in life, even in old age. But things didn't turn out nice. They turned out terrible.

When my mother got Alzheimer's, I told God and the church good-bye. I figured if there was a God he could have prevented it. And if God didn't allow it to happen, maybe he caused it to happen. So who needed him.

It's so easy to blame God, especially if he's responsible for everything. I have a convenient place to put my anger: God's to blame. God's at fault. It has taken me years to get over my anger.

Why *doesn't* God do something about Alzheimer's disease? Why does he allow it to happen in the first place? Isn't God supposed to be good?

There's one school of thought that says you shouldn't argue about the nature of God when a person is sick or dying. But when we are seriously or terminally ill or when someone we love is suffering or dying, that's the time we struggle most with the question of God's existence, God's goodness, God's power. In reality, it's a time when many of our beliefs about God are tried and tested, formed and reformed.

My own struggles with the goodness of God revolved as much around my own frustrated plans and desires as they did around my mother's disease and the devastating effects it had on both her and my father. For me, it wasn't so much an issue of the goodness of God in general as it was the goodness of God in particular. I suspect this is true for most of us.

When things are going well for us (by our standards) we may rarely question God's goodness. God's goodness only becomes an issue when we're faced with a personal crisis. Why, God, don't you do something for *my* loved one? Why don't you do something for *me?*

The answer to these questions is the same for all of us. God has already done something for us. Our job is to set aside our anger long enough to hear about it.

I believe three of the ways God speaks are through the church, through prayer, and through the Bible. Yet these are the three things we often avoid when we're angry at God, because they all involve communication with him. Communication is difficult for angry people.

The *church* is not just a building. It's a gathering of people, who hold a common belief in Jesus Christ, and who come together to worship God. The church can help us put our own situation in perspective. It can help us realize we're not alone in our grief. Others walk that road too, others who have concluded that even though they don't know all the answers, God has not abandoned them. Worshiping God with others can remind us of that fact.

> I was angry at God for several years after my mother was diagnosed with Alzheimer's disease. Then I started going back to church. I decided to go for the sake of the kids, not so much because I'd gotten over my anger. The first day back, I saw a woman whose son had been killed in a plane crash and a woman in her thirties whose husband had died of a heart attack. I realized that though they'd been through all that suffering, they still believed in God. I started crying. I cried through the whole service. That's what brought me back to God.

Prayer is simply talking with God. But talking, let alone the give-and-take of real communication, can be a difficult if not impossible task when we're angry.

If we need assistance in this area, the Bible can help. The psalmists, Job, and some of the prophets, like Jeremiah, were a lot like us. They all wrestled with the "why" questions very personally in relation to sickness and even death. They cried out to God in their confusion. We can identify with what they felt, and they, in turn, can help us express our anger and formulate our questions to God. We shouldn't feel guilty doing so.

Bernard Mobbs shared the following thoughts about expressing anger at God, especially repressed anger that often manifests itself in depression, another emotion common to caregivers:

It is significant that many of the psalmists and other Biblical writers felt free to challenge God in a way that seems highly impious to our modern sensibilities. "Wilt Thou be to me a deceitful brook, like waters that fail?" asked Jeremiah. It is reported that Teresa of Avila once said to God, "It is no wonder You have so few friends if You treat them all in this way." When a relationship is deeply loving such honesty is possible. Is it because our relationship to God is less real that we assume such a guarded manner in His presence? Certainly such superficiality does not enable us to come to terms with our true selves.[3]

It is okay to be angry at God. It is not good to stay angry forever. Christopher Allison, in *Guilt, Anger, and God*, wrote about this need to move beyond anger in our prayers and in our worship:

It is strange that the cultural taboo against admitting anger toward God has crept into the church and made us regard it as shocking and something to be suppressed. The thought of expressing our anger toward God in worship is scandalous to many. Yet this is an indication of how far we have departed from scriptural guides. The Psalms, by which Christian people have always worshipped, are generously sprinkled with anger toward God for injustice on earth. Anger certainly is a major theme in the book of Job. . . . Our sickness is our destructive anger. Our medicine is God's taking our anger. If we do not give it to him we are not healed of it. We are in bondage to our anger and are not free until our resentment is buried in him.[4]

Pain and suffering are not part of God's original plan. Disease and death were not part of the good world he created. But the original plan got flawed. God didn't cause it, but he allowed it to happen by giving us the gift called free will.

Free will means that people are not mindless robots. We can make choices. One of those choices is to love and obey God or not to love and obey him. In the beginning of the history of the human race, Adam and Eve chose not to do so. In Genesis 2–3, God commanded them in the Garden of Eden not to eat the fruit of the tree of the knowledge of good and evil. They disobeyed. The result was the entrance of suffering and death into what had been a good and perfect world.

The good news is that this world is not the end of the line. Jesus' death and resurrection remind us of that. The world will one day be set free from its suffering. Free from disease. Free from sin.

Those with Alzheimer's and those who care for them can cling to the promises God gives us in the Bible. He is working all things together for good. This is not a promise that we'll necessarily be delivered from this present suffering, but that *we have someone to walk through it with us* (see Romans 8:28 and Isaiah 42:3). No matter how hotly our anger may burn, God will never abandon us. Our anger doesn't have to consume us.

Anger at Others

As Alzheimer's takes its toll on our emotions, we will be tempted to lash out at those around us, venting our anger at the expense of other people. To keep our cool, we may need to think about safety valves.

A safety valve releases excess pressure. Steam boilers have them. When pressure inside the boiler becomes more than the pot can bear, an automatic valve on top releases the steam.

Caregivers need safety valves too. We need to know how to release our anger and frustration in *constructive* ways. We also may need to plan for the future and take preventive measures at the start to keep the pressure from building to explosive levels. Excessive pressure buildup for the caregiver can result in explosions of uncontrolled anger.

A couple of helpful emergency stopgaps for immediate situations may include the following.

➤ When tempted to verbally or even physically lash out at your loved one, pull yourself together and count to ten. If necessary, walk away from the situation. If you need to vent your anger, pound a pillow, clean out a closet, scrub a floor, chop wood. Avoid throwing and kicking things. Caregiving is expensive enough without having to replace the furniture.

➤ Put yourself in your loved one's situation. Ask yourself, "How would I like to be treated?"

In less volatile situations, distraction is a useful tool we can use with Alzheimer's sufferers and ourselves. Distraction is anything that gives mental amusement, relaxation, or diversion.

Laughing at a situation instead of getting angry or frustrated can be one way of lessening pressure and a means of distraction. You're laughing not at your loved one, but at the situation. Laughter lets off steam. Your loved one may also appreciate a good laugh at times. I laughed with my mother a lot. I think it helped us both to remember that life was not meant to be gloom and doom; it's meant to be lived and enjoyed, even the difficult moments.

Another method of coping with angry feelings is described in the New Testament. Apparently there were some angry people in the church in the city of Philippi. In Philippians, the apostle Paul's letter to that church, Paul encouraged two of the women to agree with one another, to reconcile their differences. Then he gave the whole church some tips on decreasing anxiety: rejoice in the Lord, be gentle, talk to God about your needs. In addition, Paul encouraged them to fill their minds with thoughts that are true, noble, right, pure, lovely, admirable, excellent, and praiseworthy (Philippians 4:4-9). All these things will bring peace of heart and peace of mind.

Martin Luther described this kind of meditation another way. He talked about letting our "thoughts go for a walk."[5] The scene before you may be one of utter chaos, but you don't have to be an internal wreck. When tempted to explode, turn your mind to some happy memory from the past or think about an anticipated event. Meditate on a verse from the Bible, a psalm, a hymn, some quality of God, like his love, his wisdom, his forgiving nature. Fill your mind with pleasant memories and messages from God.

When tempted to lash out at other loved ones, such as relatives who never call or visit, think about the possible reasons for their actions. Are they, too, having difficulty dealing with their loved one's illness? Do they need you to reach out to them and "give them permission" to share their own feelings of grief? Talking to your relatives about your feelings may be the best thing you can do for you both. And if talking's not possible, forgive. Carrying a load of resentment inside will be only destructive.

If nursing-home staff or other health professionals do things or say things that anger us, we should let them know about it. Not by exploding in rage, but by talking to them about their attitude, their behavior, the things we believe are negative responses.

Sometimes, because of our own guilt, we may overreact and get angry about things that are normal for nursing-home life. At other times, our anger may be justified. Others may need help in viewing the situation through your eyes, the eyes of a caregiver. We all need to be sensitive to each other and to work together as a team. Honest, open communication can help make this possible.

There are also a number of preventive measures we can take to make the buildup of anger less of a problem. Because these measures are also good cures for depression, they are covered in the following chapter.

Anger at Alzheimer's

It's normal to be angry at Alzheimer's. It's a thief, a murderer, a destroyer of minds. While ranting and raving at it won't do anyone any good, there are positive things we can do to help us feel more in command of this seemingly uncontrollable disease. We can channel our anger in practical ways by getting involved in the fight against Alzheimer's and other related dementias.

You may feel, as a caregiver, that you have neither the time nor the emotional or physical energy needed for involvement on any other level than an occasional support group meeting. If you do have the energy, however, here are a few suggestions. Some can be done individually, others with a group.

➤ Help plan a local or area seminar to educate other caregivers, health professionals, and the general public about Alzheimer's.

Your own support group could join with others in your region or plan with local hospitals, nursing schools or community service agencies.

➤ Order a box of supplies from the Alzheimer's Association and set up a table or booth to distribute them at community health fairs and county fairs. Your office on aging may also have information on Alzheimer's. Some other good resources for literature are found in appendix A.

➤ Develop and distribute a newsletter for your county or area if none is available.

➤ Offer yourself as a speaker to nursing homes, hospitals, college classes on aging and health, civic groups, and churches. This could be a formal presentation, a simple question-and-answer session, or a panel presentation.

➤ Ask a reporter from a local newspaper to write an article about Alzheimer's or submit one yourself. Raise public awareness of the disease and let people know what's available in the community.

➤ Support the Alzheimer's Association financially. Many caregivers also encourage giving a lasting memorial gift to the Association at the time of the death of a loved one.

➤ Get involved politically. Be informed about state and national legislation related to caregiving issues and funding for Alzheimer's research. Write letters to people in Congress or members of your state legislature asking their support for various bills. Attend hearings at the local and state level when aging or health issues are discussed. Offer your opinions in writing or by giving public testimony. Remember that the people who hold the purse strings at all levels of government need to hear from the people who know about the disease. The people most in the know are caregivers.

Most worthy causes became causes because someone got angry. A loved one was killed by a drunk driver, abducted from a school yard, died of cancer, or suffered from Alzheimer's disease. The war against Alzheimer's is far from over. We all need to get involved in some battles and channel our anger in constructive ways.

Chapter 14

Joy in the Mourning

"Be merciful to me, O Lord, for I am in distress; my eyes grow weak with sorrow, my soul and my body with grief. My life is consumed by anguish and my years by groaning; my strength fails because of my affliction, and my bones grow weak." David, the author of these words from Psalm 31, was depressed.

Depression is an emotion we all experience as caregivers. It can range from sadness to profound sorrow, sometimes accompanied by physical symptoms. It is triggered by many things.

Facing Depression

Depression can descend like a weight when we realize that we are no longer known by our loved one.

> They say it gets easier but I don't believe it. Each time I go to see my wife it gets harder for me. It's as if I were a total stranger. I hug her and kiss her and talk to her, but she doesn't know me. She doesn't know what's going on.

Depression can also be related to the death of expectations. Many who seem to have a bright and productive future suddenly see that future destroyed by a diagnosis.

> The real irony was that a week after my father was diagnosed, he got a letter from a company he used to work for asking him if he'd consider being the executive director.

Depression can be related to the fact that our loved one is not able to experience the joys of grandparenting.

> If I would start crying, my son would toddle upstairs, get some tissue, come sit on my lap, and pat me as if to say everything would be okay. The fact that my mother had this beautiful little grandchild who was comforting *me* because of *her* made my depression worse. I wanted so much for them to know each other, but I knew it could never happen.

Caregiver depression is often related to the anxiety, suffering, and depression our loved ones are experiencing. Their confusion doesn't eliminate emotions like fear and frustration. They also may have a sense of meaninglessness and have suicidal thoughts that can be accompanied by actions.

> I've had people say to me, especially nurses, "Don't worry about your father. You're suffering more than he is." I cannot believe that. I see my father's emotions. I see his facial expressions and his behavior. I say to myself, no one can tell me he's not feeling something.
>
> I don't believe that he's living in his own peaceful little world and that he doesn't know anything or anybody and he's not suffering. I see signs of anxiety and frustration. I see the look on his face when he wants to say something and can't get the words out. I will never be convinced he's not suffering some.

> My wife used to have a tremendous will, not wanting to let anything get the best of her. Then, just before Christmas, she gave up.

> In the spring my husband tried to commit suicide. He got out one night when I was asleep. When I woke up, I called the

police and we went searching. We finally found him up on the railroad tracks. There was a train coming. He said to the police, "Leave me alone. Leave me alone. I want to die. I have a right to kill myself if I want to."

Sometimes when we're depressed, the underlying problem is really our anger. One common definition of depression is "anger turned inward."

For months I was depressed. Months. My wife finally said to me, "Honey, I don't think your problem is depression. I think you're just angry at what happened to your father." She was right.

Searching for the Light

In his chapter on depression and loneliness in *Good Grief*, Granger Westberg likens depression to a dreadfully dark day when the sun is blacked out by clouds. He relates that people will always say, "The sun isn't shining today." But that's not true. The sun is shining, even when it appears not to be. Get on a plane, climb through the layer of clouds, and eventually you'll see that the sun *is* shining. And someone will always make the remark, says Westberg, "Too bad the people downstairs can't see this."[1]

The sunshine. The light moments. We need to look for those light moments in our loved ones' lives and not be afraid to enjoy them.

We have our jokes, our light moments. We laugh at some of the things Dad does. He's very funny sometimes. Like the day he set off the fire alarm in the nursing home. Or the day he decided to take a walk outside. He wheeled another resident out the door too. The other man didn't want to go and was hollering "No, no, no," and carrying on. But Dad didn't care. It was a nice day for a trip.

Dad always had this affectionate way of patting you on the behind. He did it to me not too long ago, and I said to Mom, "There, he's his old self. He did it again."

These little, light moments may last only a split second, but when they do appear they're good. They're very good.

Looking for the light moments is one way caregivers cope with depression. Another way is through preventive measures that may not eliminate depression for us and our loved ones, but can lighten the emotional load. They are also good ways to prevent the pressure from building up in our lives.

Maintaining Physical Fitness

If you spend half your day running around the neighborhood in search of loved ones or running up and down stairs ensuring their safety, you may be physically fit. Not all of us do this. Some loved ones are confined to wheelchairs and lead very sedentary lives. So do some caregivers.

The benefits of exercise in relation to stress reduction are well documented. When our large muscles are exercised, our involuntary muscles also relax. Stress is reduced. We have more energy. We feel better all over.

For me and several other caregivers I interviewed, swimming is a key to tension reduction. It helps ease depression and is a good way of keeping aerobically fit.

When I became a full-time caregiver, I thought my year-round swimming days might be over. The nearby lake was perfect for summer swimming, but the winter months loomed dark and dreary. Then I spoke with the director of our local YMCA. "Swim here," he said. "Your mom can come too."

Mom's "going to the Y" consisted of sitting downstairs in a deep and comfortable chair next to the television and the front desk where there was always someone in attendance. I gently restrained her with a jacket vest. She normally didn't try to wander, but I wanted to be safe rather than sorry.

Mom was very content looking through or ripping pages out of old magazines until I returned. She also seemed to enjoy the children who ran around and sometimes stopped to talk to her. Any anger or depression I had going into the pool diminished or disappeared altogether after half an hour of laps.

Some caregivers hire in-home help if they aren't able to take their loved ones with them. Some have even learned to swim and have met new friends.

If you're a runner, find a field or a track and take your loved one with you. Let her or him sit and watch you huff and puff. A wheelchair ride around the block a few times can also be good exercise for you and a good outing for your loved one. (Check with your local home-care supply store for types of chairs best suited for this. Many are very sturdy and very portable as well. Sometimes this expense is at least partially reimbursable.)

Golfing is another sport many caregiving couples have engaged in in the dementia-free past. If so, don't think you have to give this up. Your loved one may enjoy riding in the golf cart or sitting in the clubhouse looking out the window (and waving to all the golfers as my mother did). One caregiver-friendly golf club enabled me to relax and enjoy a round of golf for several summers when Mom was past the wandering stage.

There is sometimes a tendency on the part of caregivers to treat their loved ones as if they were physically ill with some disease that confines them to their homes; while this may be necessary during certain stages of Alzheimer's, it is usually not the case for all stages. Caregivers need encouragement to get up and get out and get on with their lives, including their loved ones in creative ways.

Some people with Alzheimer's can continue to enjoy golf, tennis, bowling, and other sports. They may no longer be able to keep score or play for as long as they used to, of course. But do continue to help them do the things they've always done for as long as they are able (if they can do them and not be frustrated by their diminished abilities).

Maintain a balanced diet. This may seem obvious, but many caregivers (myself included) don't do it. A balanced diet for us includes food from the basic four food groups, the same as a balanced diet for our loved ones. (See chapter eight.)

In addition, the American Heart Association recommends the following to help us look better, feel better, and be less fatigued and depressed:

- Eat foods low in saturated fats and cholesterol (fruits, vegetables, cereals, pasta, low-fat dairy products, fish, poultry, and lean meats).

- Limit salt intake by ignoring the saltshaker and avoiding highly salted, processed foods.
- Cut calories if needed to attain and maintain your weight at recommended levels.

Try to get adequate rest. The child's prayer that begins "Now I lay me down to sleep" may be only wishful thinking for a lot of caregivers, but lack of sleep does play a part in depression. If you have sleepless nights and dreary days, consider hiring an aide for at least one of those nights so you can catch up.

Keeping Mentally and Emotionally Balanced

There are a number of things we can do to help us keep our own minds engaged and our emotions on an even keel.

➤ Develop your sense of humor. One caregiver made the statement, "I think people that don't have a sense of humor are the people that are really in trouble emotionally." Do appreciate those lighter moments in your loved one's life. Try reminiscing about the good, fun, and funny times you've had together.

Get acquainted with authors who know the human condition and who can write about it with humor and wisdom, such as Garrison Keillor and Erma Bombeck. Subscribe to a magazine such as *Reader's Digest* or *Guideposts*. Read articles that can touch your heart and lift your spirits. Listen to books on tape.

There's a proverb in the Bible that says, "Even in laughter the heart may ache." We might also say that even in depression the heart may laugh. Without laughter, hearts can shrivel up and die.

➤ Maintain old hobbies and interests or develop new ones. Don't give up on the things you've enjoyed doing in the past—woodworking, reading, gardening, going to concerts, watching movies. Incorporate your loved one into your activities, if you can, or hire help for an hour or so each week (or find a volunteer) so you can get out and pursue your interests. That's a part of maintaining mental health. Both you and your loved one will be richer for it.

➤ A wheelchair can also be a worthwhile investment, not only for exercise but simply for going places. Even if your loved one is still able to walk well, wheelchairs can be useful for situations that require longer, more tiring walks.

With the aid of a wheelchair, I was able to take my mother Christmas shopping, to the zoo, to museums and parades, and even camping at a state park equipped with cabins and nature trails designed for the disabled.

Check with your Department of Motor Vehicles or County Clerk about acquiring a handicap-vehicle sticker or card for your car. You will probably need one, even if your loved one is ambulatory and doesn't require a wheelchair. A physician will have to sign a statement of need; it's well worth the phone call, stamp, or office visit to obtain it.

➤ If music has been an important part of your loved one's life as well as your own, don't underestimate its value. Often the ability to play a musical instrument is still retained, though memory for other things is lost. Attend musical events together for as long as possible.

➤ Maintain relationships with other people or develop new relationships. You may find it impossible to go out much, but you can invite people in. Don't feel they wouldn't want to come. Most people enjoy being invited out to eat. Suggest they bring a dish to pass if your budget is tight. This may be a good way to get to know other caregivers, too, and provide an evening out for all concerned.

➤ If depression is a chronic or severe problem over which you seem to have little control, you may need to seek professional assistance. There are many trained counselors in private practice and local mental health clinics available with counselors on staff. Members of the clergy can also be good sources of support and are usually well acquainted with depression. Sometimes medication may be needed as well as counseling.

Signs and symptoms of a more severe depression can include:

- generalized weakness/fatigue
- uncontrollable or frequent episodes of crying
- weight loss or, sometimes, weight gain
- low blood pressure
- headache or generalized aches and pains
- constipation
- sleep disturbances
- memory lapses or confusion
- symptoms of anxiety: tightness in the chest, stomach cramps, shaking, dizziness, a lump in the throat, sweating, diarrhea, heart palpitations
- excessive drinking
- mood swings that range from euphoric to depressive
- negative self-concept; low self-esteem
- suicidal thoughts

Seeking Spiritual Support

Spiritual support for both you and your loved one can take many forms. One of the best support systems is a local church.

Church, of all places, should be a place where you can take your loved one even in times of bizarre behavior. Church families that are sensitive to the needs of memory-impaired people and their caregivers will be able to come up with some creative ways to help you both enjoy various aspects of the worship experience, whether on a Sunday morning or at various times throughout the week. If you don't find this to be true, talk to the pastor. You may have to make your needs known directly. You may also find you have to shop around a bit for a church that meets your needs. Finding a good church can be a little like finding a good home-care worker. Sooner or later, with persistence and prayer, you'll find the perfect match.

One church I know of gives caregivers a break each Sunday by offering free home care. People in the church take turns sitting for a woman's husband, who is memory-impaired, so she can attend services. Another sponsors various caregiver support groups and offers training seminars on topics related to caregiving.

When I got over my own anger at God and was looking for a church, I knew for certain when I had found the perfect match. This knowledge hit me one Sunday when, in the middle of the pastor's sermon, the congregation began singing "Home on the Range."

The reason for the song was an elderly man named Hoppy, who suffered from dementia. Every Sunday the pastor's words would trigger something else in Hoppy's memory that related to a familiar song.

This particular Sunday the pastor was talking about going to our heavenly home. The mention of "home" was all Hoppy needed to break into a chorus of "Home on the Range." The pastor just smiled and encouraged the congregation to join in. So we all stood and sang. This, I thought, is a group of people who are comfortable with people with dementia!

Westberg wrote about the church as a place of healing, a place where our spirits can be lifted, and where the depressed can truly see the sunshine through the clouds:

> A congregation of religious people ought to live up to the well-known description of "the community of the concerned." If they are actually concerned about those who mourn, who feel lost from the world and from God, then they will earn the lasting gratitude of those who mourn.[2]

For my mother and me, this was true of the church we attended. It has also been true for many other caregivers.

Spiritual support can also come from another source—God himself.

Finding God in the Wilderness

Depression has often been called "a wilderness experience." Many Alzheimer's sufferers know this to be true. They become lost in their own confusion and the tangled web of their minds. In the book *My Journey into Alzheimer's Disease*, Robert Davis, a Presbyterian minister diagnosed with Alzheimer's, wrote about one aspect of his own wilderness experience:

I go to church services to worship God, but I cannot sing. I cannot join in the readings or prayers because my mind cannot do two things at once. Singing and group readings take several processes going on at once to listen to the others and pace my reading in time with theirs. Such a simple thing. But impossible for me now.

Suddenly I stand out in the worship service, silent and continually confused during the time of hymn singing. I feel that my fellow worshipers are looking at me askance, wondering why I do not join in. My newfound paranoia also sets in, making me wonder if they think by my silence I am showing disapproval of the hymn, the church, the musicians, or the people around me. This time of joy has been changed into a time of frustration and anxiety.

Now I would like to come into the service late, after the singing of the first hymns or any responsive reading. However, out of propriety I do not. How I long to again sing my heart out and thus fully express my joy, but I cannot. The sorrow of this and this sense of loss fills me so much that often tears come to my eyes—tears that only compound my paranoia and my ever-present fears of what people are thinking.[3]

As caregivers we also experience the empty, barren wilderness as we gradually lose our loved one to a disease. As one caregiver asked, "Where is the *essence* of my father?" The essence. Those indispensable, unique characteristics that make our loved one our loved one. Where are they? They're gradually lost with the progression of Alzheimer's disease, leaving us in a wilderness tinged with the memories of the past.

Elisabeth Elliot, in her book *Loneliness*, wrote the following: "The wildernesses spoken of in the Bible were usually very barren places, but God can change that. He can make streams in the desert, springs in the valley, and furnish tables in the wilderness."[4]

The streams, the springs, the tables that God can create can turn our loneliness and depression into a deep, abiding experience of joy. This joy comes as we are able to accept our circumstances and let God meet and care for us in the midst of them. God alone can deliver us from our wilderness of mourning and turn our sorrow into joy. "I will turn their mourning into gladness; I will give them comfort and joy instead of sorrow" (Jeremiah 31:13).

Finding Joy

My mother used to call me Sharon. Then it became "Honey," the name she called me as a child. Pretty soon I became "Mom" to her as her Alzheimer's progressed. And finally I became "Gramma."

For most people life is filled with roles. For caregivers, it's also filled with role-reversals.

> Just when I thought the nest was empty, I find it filled again. Not with grandchildren, but with my husband.

> I see the role change with both my parents as I handle their affairs. I handle everything for them. I'm their mouthpiece, their spokesperson. As soon as I moved back home, my mother saw me as the one in charge.
>
> But I never looked on my parents as children. I just believe that now, in their senior years, they need more help. And I can help them. I prayed for years, when I was away from home, that God would give me an opportunity to care for my parents in their old age if they needed it. I've accepted it and am thankful for it.

If we are not able to accept the role-reversal as part of God's plan for our lives, we're never going to be able to experience true joy. The role of a caregiver can be a blessing or a curse, depending on our attitude. It can help us mature and blossom or it can cause us to wither away and die, emotionally and spiritually. It can bring us closer to God or it can drive a wedge between us.

Yet we are not the only ones experiencing a role-reversal. Our loved ones are too. Robert Davis shares his own perceptions of the losses he experienced:

In my rational moments I am still me. Alzheimer's disease is like a reverse aging process. Having drunk from the fountain of youth one is caught in the time tunnel without a stopping place at the height of beauty and strength. Cruelly, it whips us back to the place of infancy. First the memories go, then perceptions, feelings, knowledge, and, in the last stage, our ability to talk and take care of our most basic human needs. Thrusting us headlong into the seventh stage of man, "without teeth, without sight, without everything."

At this stage, while I still have some control of thoughts and feelings, I must learn to take on the role of the infant in order to make use of whatever gifts are left to me.[5]

Davis, unlike many people with Alzheimer's, was able to write about his feelings of loss. His book, written with his wife, Betty, is a moving account of one man's journey into Alzheimer's, written by a man with a deep faith in God. God meets him in the wilderness. He gives him joy.

For Robert Davis, the supreme joy comes in his relationship with Jesus and the knowledge of Jesus' love for him. Joy, too, comes in a deep, abiding faith that this world is not the end of things. There is a place called heaven, and he fully intends to go there:

Perhaps the journey that takes me away from reality into the blackness of that place of the blank, emotionless, unmoving Alzheimer's stare is in reality a journey into the richest depths of God's love that few have experienced on earth. Who can know what goes on deep inside a person who is so withdrawn? At that time, I will be unable to give you a clue, but perhaps we can talk about it later in the timeless joy of heaven. On second thought, all these heartaches won't really matter over there, will they?[6]

All these heartaches won't matter in the future. And as we let Jesus touch our own lives and our loved ones' lives here on earth, they won't matter as much in the present. Because Jesus, after all, is joy.

Part Four

SAYING GOOD-BYE

The last enemy to be destroyed is death.

1 Corinthians 15:26

Chapter 15

The Difficult Decisions

"There is a time for everything," wrote the author of Ecclesiastes, "and a season for every activity under heaven" (Ecclesiastes 3:1). Many of us will relinquish primary caregiving for a season of institutionalization. For others, a season of caregiving at home will culminate in the death of a loved one. Neither change is easy; both bring a host of difficult decisions.

Knowing When to Institutionalize

It's time. Those two words are charged with a bushel full of conflicting emotions for caregivers who have finally made the decision to institutionalize their loved one. The decision never comes easily.

> My husband had been crying a lot. He kept saying, "Help me, help me, please help me," over and over again. Nobody in the house was sleeping. Every day the furniture was turned upside down. He urinated in the middle of the kitchen. On weekends we just didn't bother with the house at all. People would come to visit and the chairs would be on top of the table. The couch was sometimes upside down. It was chaos.
> Then one day I got a call at work. My husband was at home, beating on the front door, crying and crying because he couldn't go out. One of the home-health aides had called me, wondering what to do. A switch went on in my mind. I said to myself, "It's time."

The right time to institutionalize is often related to the realization that we are no longer physically able to care for our loved one because of our own health problems.

> I've heard people say "I would never put my father or mother in a nursing home." Well, I wouldn't have either if I could have handled him at home. But I couldn't. My mother couldn't. Physically we just couldn't handle it.
>
> You have to be practical. You have to realize when you simply can't cope anymore—physically or emotionally.
>
> When you can no longer give the people you love most the care they should have, that's when you have to decide.

> I had help for eight hours a day prior to putting my husband in a nursing home. That still wasn't enough. I was up all night, every night. And I'm eighty-eight years old.
>
> It got to the point where I knew it was either him or me, and I knew I wasn't ready for a nursing home yet.

Physical violence by our loved one may lead to the event that triggers institutionalization.

> One morning my husband hit me on the shoulder. He'd threatened me a good number of times, but he'd never actually done it before. It didn't really hurt, but it scared me.
>
> Just then the phone rang. It was my daughter. I was crying as I told her what had happened. She immediately called the social-service worker who was already providing some home-care help for us. The social worker came to see me that afternoon. That was a Monday. On Thursday my husband was admitted to the nursing home, one fairly close to our home.
>
> I was glad he was going to that particular home. I'd visited it once before and liked it the best of any of them. That made the decision a little easier.

For others, safety may be the trigger issue—safety for our loved one and other family members.

> Daddy kept falling. We tried to prevent it, but the only way was to keep restrained in a chair, and he fought that so. The other alternative was to sedate him, but then it was impossible for me to physically handle him. So we finally decided that, for his sake and mine, the nursing home was best.

> The day my mother set the wastebasket on fire in the bedroom was the day we decided to do something. She just wasn't safe anymore.

So circumstances make us decide. Yet we still have to deal with our tangled emotions. And the predominant emotion is guilt. Often, guilt surfaces because of others' attitudes.

> There are so many people who think you put your parents in a nursing home because you want to get rid of them, that you don't want to be bothered, that you no longer care, that you don't appreciate what they did for you. They don't realize those are not the reasons at all.

Fortunately, the initial guilt is often followed by relief; based on our situation, we have made the best decision for all concerned. Don't be surprised, however, if ambivalent feelings remain.

> Mom still feels guilty at times, but she knows Dad is getting good care. Mom really does worry about him. She prays for him every day. And I take her to see him once a week. She's prepared, if anything happens, to accept it.

We might be distressed if Dad were anyplace else but the home he's in. It's good, it's clean, and it's close. They're kind to him there. The doctor comes in every Friday and goes over his record and visits with him. The doctor's on call if there's a problem.

All things considered, it's the best we could ask for.

There was a lot of guilt. The nursing home was the last place I ever wanted Daddy to go. When I went to visit him, I'd sit in the car and pray for strength to go in and go through all the conflicting emotions I knew I'd have. I'd pray that I could act cheerful.

That first week I just wanted to pack Daddy up and take him home. I even thought of quitting my job to take care of him. But, even while I was thinking about it, I knew I couldn't. I knew it wasn't the best. For me. For my family. For Daddy.

I still feel guilty whenever I visit my wife. The other night I went to see her and she hugged me and kissed me and seemed to know who I was. I cried. I couldn't help it.

But when she is not good and doesn't know me and doesn't pay any attention to me, I'm glad she's where she is.

So I'm up. And I'm down.

I do feel guilty because I don't get to the nursing home as often as I used to. In the beginning I saw my father every other day. But then I suddenly realized there are other things that need to be taken care of.

My mother, who's still at home, has needs too. Lots of them. I'm running her house too. She can live alone but she can't do her own cooking. I cook at home and make up frozen dinners for her.

I'm simply not always able to get up, get out, and go see my father every day.

We may wonder, "Did I make the right decision?" But the day will come when we know certainly the answer is yes.

In the beginning it was hard. Dad always wanted to come home with us. When it was time for us to leave, we'd say to the nurses, "Please get Dad's attention." And the nurses would try to distract him while we snuck out.

Then one day when we were getting ready to go, Dad turned to us and said, "You know, girls, this isn't a bad place. I rather like it. I think I'll buy it."

All of a sudden, our guilt about institutionalization was gone.

In the midst of this difficult decision making, some caregivers long for the good old days, an era when life was simple and families stayed together through thick and thin. Nancy Mace and Peter Rabins, in *The 36-Hour Day*, put the good old days in perspective:

We tend to think of the "good old days" as a time when families took care of their elderly at home. In fact, in the past not many people lived long enough for their families to be faced with the burden of caring for a person with a demential illness. The people who did become old and sick were in their fifties and sixties and the sons and daughters who cared for them were considerably younger than you may be when your parent needs care in his seventies and eighties. Today many "children" of an ailing parent are themselves in their sixties or seventies.[1]

Times have changed. For today's families, the first goal is to support a loved one in whatever environment best meets his or her needs.

The second goal is to rid ourselves of the guilt that comes when nursing-home placement is necessary. It may help to remember that up to sixty percent of nursing-home beds are filled with people who suffer from Alzheimer's disease or a related dementia. We are not alone.

What Are the Options?

Institutionalization does not solely refer to nursing homes. There are a number of options available for caregiving away from home.

The Adult Home. The adult home is designed for people who don't require regular medical or nursing care, but who cannot live alone because of age, poor health, or a chronic disability. Availability and license status will vary. Most are run as businesses by people concerned for the elderly and disabled. Not all homes will accept people with Alzheimer's. On the other hand, more and more people are opening their homes exclusively to Alzheimer's sufferers. However, not all will accept or keep people when they become totally disabled and need more intensive nursing care.

Check around. Talk with other caregivers. Many families prefer this option because of the homey atmosphere and personal attention given to loved ones.

Payment varies. Licensed homes may accept Medicare (under certain circumstances), Medicaid, and/or Supplemental Social Security. Private, unlicensed homes are generally private-pay only, though they are usually much cheaper than nursing homes.

Nursing Homes. There are various types of nursing homes. Some are considered *proprietary,* which means they expect to make a profit. Others are *nonproprietary,* or nonprofit. They are run by families, corporations, churches, denominations, and community agencies. Nonprofit, public nursing homes are generally county run.

Quality varies from home to home and has little to do with a home's profit or nonprofit status. Based on my own experience, quality depends on the training and attitudes of the personnel.

Nursing homes can provide a skilled or an intermediate level of care. Usually these two levels are combined in one facility on two or more separate units. One advantage of placing a loved one in such a home is that they should be able to transfer easily to another unit—rather than to another nursing home—should a change in care be required.

Special-Care Units. Some hospitals and nursing homes have special-care units for people with dementia. These are usually secured wards that allow people to freely wander in a supervised environment. Your regional chapter of the Alzheimer's Association may be a good resource for specific information.

Shopping for a Nursing Home

There are many things to consider when shopping for a nursing home. The following points may help make things easier.

➤ Talk to other caregivers who have placed loved ones with Alzheimer's in nursing homes. How did they choose that particular home? Are they happy with it?

➤ Seek out nurses, social workers, or others in your community who work with the elderly (specifically with Alzheimer's sufferers). Ask what's available in the area.

➤ Keep your own limitations and the concerns of family in mind. For instance, there may be an excellent home several hours away that has a special unit for people with Alzheimer's. Is this an option? Would visitation by family and friends still be possible?

➤ Meet with your loved one's physician. It's good to have a doctor involved early in the planning process, for information and support. Also, a physician's referral will usually be needed for admission to a nursing home.

Unfortunately, many caregivers shop for a nursing home as they shop for Christmas presents: at the last minute.

This is unwise. Plan ahead. This will enable you to choose the home best suited to your loved one's personality and needs. Don't wait for a crisis and then expect a bed to be available. Chances are, it won't.

Reasons for advance planning include the following:

Waiting lists. Some homes have them, others don't. Even if you're unsure about placement, it's wise to fill out an application at a number of homes. (You can always say no if you are called and are not ready to place. Just ask the home to call you again in the future.) Sometimes many months go by before a bed is available. With hospitals discharging patients quicker and sicker, some homes are more likely to admit directly from the hospital itself.

Some homes limit the number of people they will admit with a demential illness. In this case, it's essential that you be placed on a waiting list.

Legal loose ends. There's always a need to explore legal issues related to nursing-home placement. It takes time to tie up loose ends. Don't shortchange yourself.

Additional Criteria

The American Health Care Association is a nonprofit organization of long-term care facilities dedicated to improving health care of the convalescent and chronically ill of all ages. Its comprehensive list of criteria to consider when choosing a nursing home can be requested by writing them at the address listed in appendix A.

In addition to using a checklist, evaluate a nursing home or any other similar facility with your own common sense and common *senses.*

Visit several facilities. Planned visits with the nursing home social workers and/or nursing-home administrators are essential, but you may also want to arrive unexpectedly, too. Talk with some of the residents and their families. Observe the residents involved in activities both social and health related. Watch the nursing-home staff at work. Pay attention to first impressions and to what your senses are telling you.

What do you *feel?* Does the place feel like a home or an institution? Even in very large homes, caring, compassionate, noninstitutional attitudes will show—if the staff have them.

What do you *see?* The best homes combine good nursing care with a homelike atmosphere. Are individual rooms cheerful, with pictures on the wall and mementoes from home? Are the majority of residents out of bed, dressed in street clothes, and well groomed? Do most appear alert? *Alert* does not necessarily mean "oriented." It has more to do with wakefulness. If the majority of residents are not alert, it may be a sign of inappropriate medication.

Do the nursing assistants (the people doing most of the hands-on care) look frenzied and frazzled or do they appear relatively calm and relaxed? Ask about the aide-to-resident ratio; you'll want to know if the home is adequately staffed.

What do you *hear*? Pay attention to what people are saying and their tone of voice. Do the staff talk to the residents? What do they talk about? Do they speak to them with dignity and respect? Don't be unduly upset if you hear residents holler or scream at times. Bath and shower times are prime occasions for this; confused residents may resent this intrusion or be frightened.

What do you *smell*? It's not possible to have a completely odor-free environment in a nursing home. You may note the smell of urine or stool coming from a room or two as you walk down the hall. This should be an exception rather than the rule. If there is a pervasive odor of urine or some other unpleasant smell, ask why. You should also see housekeeping staff mopping and damp dusting.

Ask the nursing director or director of training what kind of training staff receive. Good homes require extensive training of all nursing assistants. You might ask to see a copy of their training manual. A good course usually lasts approximately one hundred hours and is generally taught over a three-week period.

Good homes also have an orientation period for staff that includes an overview of residents' rights; issues of resident abuse, mistreatment and neglect; the problems of aging; fire safety for staff and residents; and training in the proper methods of lifting and moving residents. Ask to see a copy of the orientation program. This will be readily available in most nursing homes.

How Do I Pay the Bills?

One of the first questions a nursing home will ask the family of a prospective resident is, Who will pay the bill? Nursing homes aren't cheap. But their high cost covers nutritious meals, your loved one's share of the rent and utilities, and medical care that involves many trained personnel.

Paying for all of those benefits can be handled in a variety of ways, including the following:

Private funds. Some families are able to pay for nursing home care privately, though not necessarily forever. Costs will vary and may increase annually.

Spouses, children, and other responsible parties will need to consult with a lawyer about their own financial liability and issues of concern. For example, are you legally and financially responsible for a parent in a nursing home? For all or part of their care? Rules vary from state to state. Talk with the nursing-home social worker, but don't sign anything until you've also checked with your own financial adviser.

Medicare. Medicare is a health-insurance program sponsored by the federal government for people over sixty-five. It may also apply to people under sixty-five, who are blind or suffer from some other disability, through a program known as Supplemental Security Income (SSI).

The Medicare rules for eligibility are complex. Generally speaking, Medicare provides the best benefits to people who are hospitalized and who would require high levels of skilled nursing care at home or in long-term care facilities following hospitalization. In the latter two cases, coverage is usually restricted to specific types of skilled nursing care, for a limited number of days. Talk with hospital staff about Medicare coverage, but don't depend on Medicare to pick up much of the tab.

Information booklets about Medicare and SSI can be obtained through your Social Security office.

Medicaid. Medicaid pays for the majority of nursing-home residents. It is a federal program administered through each state. The name *Medicaid* may differ from state to state. Application is through your local social-services department or department of welfare. Applying can be a time-consuming process, and it is one more reason for starting the application process early.

Again, speak with a lawyer who is well versed in Medicaid regulations and health needs of the elderly.

Insurance and pensions. Private health insurance and certain life insurance and pension plans may also cover some nursing-home costs. Some plans are excellent, while others pay negligible amounts for custodial-type care. Talk directly with your insurance agent or a company representative about available benefits.

Veteran benefits. If your loved one is a veteran or the spouse of a veteran, check with the Veterans Administration about benefits. There are usually some veterans' hospitals or nursing homes in each state as well. Speak with them directly about medical and financial eligibility.

Making That Difficult Decision

As you weigh the pros and cons of placement, consider the following issues and questions. Your responses should help you make a wise and appropriate decision based on your loved one's needs and the needs of your family.

Health. Can you continue to care for your loved one at home without jeopardizing your own mental, emotional, and physical health? What about the health of other family members? Is the care you're able to provide keeping your loved one as healthy as possible—or is ill health increasing in frequency, duration, or intensity?

Safety. Can you continue to provide a safe environment, or are accidents increasingly beyond your control? Is the safety of the rest of the family at risk if your loved one remains at home?

Support. Do you have enough support from family, friends, and community service providers to handle increasing care needs? Is the help you need (or will need) affordable as well as available?

Placing my own mother in a nursing home was not an easy decision for me. I was one of those people who had always told myself, "I'll never do it." But then, one day, I did, just like other caregivers have done. Health, safety, and support were all factors in making the decision. It seemed that Mom and I were spending more and more time on the floor; she was no longer able to walk as the Alzheimer's progressed into the final stages, and transfers from chair to bed or wheelchair to car were becoming increasingly difficult. Safety for both of us was an issue coupled with dwindling finances and a decision I had made to move to another city to continue my education. Mom's unexpected trip to the hospital for a condition unrelated to her Alzheimer's was the trigger event that convinced me that "now was the time." Friends and relatives were supportive, realizing better than I that home care was not really providing the best for her, no matter how well I thought I was coping.

Continuing to Care

As many caregivers (including myself) have testified, you can still care for a loved one in practical ways after he or she moves to a nursing home. Relinquishment does not mean abandonment. In fact, a good home will welcome any support you can offer. This includes visits as well as helpful hints—drawn from your years of experience—about caring for your loved one.

➤ People who are confused do better in familiar surroundings. Suggest arranging the furniture as it was at home, if this is possible. Some homes will even allow you to bring in familiar furniture. Also bring pictures, photographs, and, of course, your loved one's favorite clothes.

➤ Be with your loved one on the day of admission. You won't necessarily need to stay all day, but several hours will be helpful for the initial transition. Take someone with you for support—another family member or a best friend. Don't assume loved ones won't adjust. Sometimes they settle in immediately; if they no longer recognize familiar faces, everyone may be family to them.

► Before or on the day of admission the social worker will want to know more about your loved one's background. This is called "taking a social history." As a nurse, I find social histories to be vitally important. The history might include the type of work your loved one used to do, places of employment, special hobbies and interests, information about children and grandchildren (including names and addresses), church affiliation and involvement, languages spoken, and so on. Unfortunately, on some charts the information is very sparse, either because there was no family to give it or because families felt the information was too personal.

The activities department of the home can use this information to plan a program suited to your loved one's needs. For example, if your loved one was very active in church, provisions can be made for attending worship services and special religious services in the home. Other activities might include social hours, in-home movies, bingo, or baking. A person with Alzheimer's may not be able to participate actively in these activities but may enjoy socializing in a group.

A social history also can be helpful for the nursing assistants caring for your loved one. Knowing something about your loved one's interests and occupation can provide a point of contact for conversation or provide the caregivers with something to talk about.

Anne Evans and John Smith exemplify the value of a detailed social history. Anne Evans was a resident in the early stages of Alzheimer's who had been very depressed. I attended one of the care conferences when the staff talked about possible reasons for her depression and suggested ways to cheer her up. Leafing through her social history, I noticed that she had been an avid golfer. I went home that night, wrapped up a new package of golf balls and brought it in the next day. Anne and I unwrapped the package together. This small action didn't cure her depression, but it brightened her day and provided a point of contact. She enjoys talking about this past interest, and that has opened the door for discussing other concerns as well.

John Smith was a resident who had been comatose for over a year. A nursing assistant told me, "I always turn his radio to a classical-music station when I take care of him. One of his relatives told me he played the violin and was in an orchestra when he was younger." That information wasn't part of Mr. Smith's social history. I added a note to the chart and we put a sign on the radio about keeping it tuned to a particular station.

These pieces of helpful information can easily be forgotten in the busyness of a loved one's admission. Feel free, though, to pass them along (preferably in writing) at any time, so they can be shared with staff members and benefit your loved one.

➤ Continued visitation is important. Some people visit daily, others weekly, others less frequently. There is no right or wrong schedule. Feel your way into a visitation schedule that meets the needs of everyone involved.

Visiting doesn't always have to be in the home. Plan to take your loved one out: go to a restaurant, have a picnic in the park, go shopping, or attend church. Going back to a previous home may or may not be an option to consider. Some people easily adjust to this; others want to stay home once they get there. Some people with Alzheimer's experience increased stress related to outings and home visits and may actually be better off remaining in the home; don't feel guilty if this is the case, even on holidays that are normally family occasions. The nursing home staff will be honest with you if you ask them about how your loved one readjusts to the home routine after a home visit.

When you do visit, use the time to care for your loved one in practical ways. Give a manicure, go for a walk or a wheelchair ride, assist with feeding at mealtime (unless nursing-home policy prohibits this). Actually doing something physical may help you feel better about the visit.

Continuing-Care Issues

Once your loved one settles in, concerns will continue to arise. Talk to the charge nurse, social worker, or director of nursing about any problems. Remember, though, that some things will be done much differently than they were at home. For example, your loved one may need to wear a vest or waist restraint when in bed or sitting up to protect against falling or injuring other residents. If you have any questions about the type or quality of care given, talk with the people in charge. Let your concerns be known.

Take advantage of home-sponsored activities that enhance staff and family relationships. This can be a less stressful time to get to know the staff more personally. Nursing homes truly are extended families in many ways. These types of activities, when everyone is really enjoying each other's company, can help you see the home as a caring community of friends.

Inevitably, questions arise concerning terminal care. If a loved one suddenly stopped breathing, what should be done? Should he or she be resuscitated? In some facilities all staff are trained in CPR (cardiopulmonary resuscitation) and would be expected to try to revive any resident suffering a cardiac or respiratory arrest. In many other homes, staff would immediately call an ambulance. The rescue squad might then attempt to resuscitate.

Most states have special laws governing resuscitation that apply to people who are terminally ill or who want to die in peace—minus any "heroic" measures. In New York State, for example, there is a "Do Not Resuscitate" law. There are forms to fill out, papers to sign, people to talk with. The nursing-home social worker should discuss this with you. Planning ahead can make things easier for you and your loved one.

Finally, stay in tune with your feelings. Be involved in a support group. Some nursing homes have support groups that regularly meet in the home. Ask about them.

Guilt, anger, and depression do not automatically disappear the day you walk through the nursing-home door, or the day you walk out and leave your loved one behind. But we can deal with all these emotions the same way we dealt with them when our loved ones were home: with support from others, help from God, and the understanding that what we're experiencing is normal. We *will* survive.

The Autopsy

My grandfather said, "No autopsy. Your grandmother's been through enough hurt already. We don't need to do that to her."

I've made plans for a brain autopsy for my father. As a matter of fact, I have a postmortem file.

When I left for vacation recently I told a friend, "Here's the file. If anything happens to Dad, get the file to my brother. He'll have to act immediately."

I have the materials filed both in the nursing home and at the hospital where Dad's doctor practices, so they'll know this is what we want.

It's a very difficult thing to plan. Just the thought of what they'll have to do hurts me terribly. But if it can help future victims—if it can help future generations of our own family—it will be worth the tears.

When I'm alone, bored, and the weather's nasty, I think about Mom's death and the autopsy. I know it had to be done.

There was the chance that they would find something in her brain that would give them a clue as to what really goes wrong. And I know my mother would have said, "Do it, if it's going to help someone else."

I was planning on having an autopsy done right up until the the time of my mother's death; then I changed my mind at the last minute.

I felt guilt about my decision at first but I don't anymore. I don't see this as a moral issue or an issue of right or wrong, but as a personal one that every relative makes based on their own particular circumstances.

Requesting a brain autopsy is a final step many caregivers decide to take, for a number of good reasons.

Brain autopsies conclusively confirm or deny the presence of Alzheimer's disease. During an autopsy, the pathologist microscopically examines sections of the brain. If Alzheimer's was present, there will be plaques and tangles, the disease's main characteristics. If Alzheimer's was the cause of the dementia, treatment for symptomatic relatives may be possible. Family members could then take advantage of experimental-drug research and medical advances if diagnosed early.

Families will want also to know if plaques and tangles are *absent*. For people worried about the disease's genetic possibilities, such news can offer relief.

The only other test that can conclusively confirm or deny Alzheimer's is a brain biopsy, performed while the patient is alive. These are rarely done. (Biopsies require both extensive samples and the subject's informed consent.)

The clinical diagnosis of Alzheimer's disease made while a person is living can be inaccurate, no matter how much testing is done. Autopsies can provide conclusive evidence.

Brain autopsies contribute to Alzheimer's research. Studying the living brain is difficult. Unlike other major organs, the brain is not easily probed. It's encased in a bony "safe" designed to protect it from infection and trauma.

The brain also has the added protection of a special membrane called the blood-brain barrier, which prevents undesirable chemicals from entering the brain. This protective sheath makes it equally difficult to withdraw any foreign chemicals from living brain tissue, chemicals that might give clues to Alzheimer's cause.

Alzheimer's is a uniquely human disease that affects our thoughts, emotions, personalities, and wills. Animal models, useful for research in many other diseases, are unsuitable for researching a disease of the mind.

Brain autopsies help generate funding for research. Funding for research for any disease is based largely on its prevalence. In the case of Alzheimer's, it's especially important that accurate statistics are gathered.

These factors highlight the importance of brain-tissue research. A cure is unlikely unless a cause is discovered, and no cause will be discovered without continuing exploration into the abnormalities of autopsied human brain cells.

Consenting to an Autopsy

Without an autopsy, physicians are usually reluctant to cite Alzheimer's disease as the cause of death. This reluctance does a disservice to you, to the memory of your loved one, and to future generations. It will only be eliminated if family members consent to autopsies.

A brain autopsy is not done automatically at the time of death. It must be requested. It is a decision that should not be left to the emotion-laden days surrounding the death of a loved one. A sudden, unexpected death could eliminate the opportunity for an autopsy because of the necessary requirements. As prepared as I thought I was, this happened with my own mother. I had moved to another part of the state and was in the process of obtaining autopsy forms when the call came from the nursing home that Mom's condition had changed for the worse. Foresight and planning are essential well before the time a crisis hits.

A great deal of information, guidance, and support is needed before a decision for an autopsy can be made. Help is available from a number of sources.

➤ Start with your local support group. Ask others in the group if they have gone through this process. Have a speaker on the subject come to a meeting and discuss the regulations that apply to your community.

➤ Think through the reasons for autopsy and weigh the pros and cons. You may have religion-based objections. Talk to your pastor, priest, or rabbi if this is a concern for you.

You may feel that your loved one's body will be desecrated or treated with disrespect. Rest assured that a brain autopsy causes no disfigurement to a person's face or body. There is no reason why, following an autopsy, you cannot have an open casket viewing or funeral.

➤ Discuss the decision with family members. If there is a surviving spouse, the ultimate decision rests with him or her. Still, it is good to agree as a family—and all family members will have an opinion on the subject, colored by their emotions and knowledge of what's involved.

➤ Send for autopsy information. A national autopsy network has been established through the Alzheimer's Association to help educate caregivers about autopsy procedures and make autopsy arrangements less stressful. Particularly helpful is a list of autopsy-network affiliate centers that is available by writing the Alzheimer's Association. Each state has a regional autopsy-network representative who will also be able to help you. Further information is in appendix A.

Making Medical Arrangements

Each hospital or research center affiliated with the autopsy network has specific written protocols or instructions. These instructions include information for the local pathologist on how to prepare the brain tissue for examination. If you want the brain tissue to be autopsied for both diagnostic and research purposes, your pathologist needs to know this; there are two separate processes involved in tissue preparation. (The Alzheimer's Association recommends both procedures.) The instructions may also include information for the family to fill out related to the history and progression of your loved one's disease.

You may also need to complete a family history form. This will include the names and health histories of living members of your loved one's family, as well as the causes of death for deceased family members. It is especially important to state whether there is any history of Alzheimer's disease or severe memory loss. Death certificates may provide this information.

The research center you choose can provide you with a packet of forms to complete. The information may include a release form giving permission for your loved one's physician to release these reports to the research facility. Copies of CT and MRI scans, EEGs, medical laboratory tests, neurological work-ups, and so on should also be sent to the research center at the time of death.

If the autopsy is done in the hospital where your loved one was diagnosed and/or treated, there will usually be no charge. If autopsied tissue is sent to another research facility, there may be a modest transportation or examination fee. This information is available from your regional representative.

Talk with your loved one's physician and the local pathologist. Don't assume your physician will make the autopsy arrangements. You will be expected to make your own arrangements and consult directly with the pathologist. Make sure the pathologist knows what to do. Give the pathologist a copy of the protocols from the research center you have chosen or request that the center send a copy.

You'll also need to make special arrangements in case your loved one should die on a weekend or holiday. A brain autopsy generally must be conducted within twelve to eighteen hours after death. Both you and the pathologist need to be aware of the specific time factor.

A competent relative with the highest legal standing (for example, a spouse) will also have to sign an autopsy permit or request form. Some states require signatures from several relatives. This form should be kept with your loved one's records. In some states you may presign this months before the actual need arises. In other states, you need to sign a permit at the time of death. In either case, a confirmation of your wishes for an autopsy will probably be required at the time of death.

Alert the hospital or nursing home about autopsy arrangements you have made. Don't assume everyone is oriented to this procedure.

Contact your funeral director. The funeral director must be involved and aware of your wishes. The body should not be embalmed before the brain is removed. (Some funeral homes resist autopsies. Make sure the home you choose will comply with your wishes.)

Knowing the Truth

Several months after the autopsy, you or your physician should receive a written, detailed explanation of the autopsy results from the neuropathologist who conducted the autopsy. This will include a diagnosis based on both large-scale and microscopic findings.

Consenting to an autopsy is never a painless decision for anyone who is a caregiver. After all the suffering our loved one has experienced, we may feel he or she is entitled to rest in peace. But if we see the autopsy as an aid to research and the ultimate diagnostic test for a disease that, someday, may be arrested, prevented, and cured, it becomes a pain that offers promise.

For us, our loved ones, and our families, the battle may soon be over. For millions of others, it has only just begun. The information gained from our loved one's autopsy may be the vital link in the chain that will one day reveal the true cause of this devastating disease.

Chapter 16

Blowing Out the Candle

Muriel sat at the kitchen table. The wick in the kerosene lantern flared, casting a warm glow over the chilled room. The storm had abated but the electricity was still out. Muriel stared at the flame, and thought about her mother's death several days earlier.

Her mother's death had been a lot like that flickering wick. A lot like the dimly burning candle that sat on the mantel in the dining room.

Death had not come easily for Ruth. Neither had life. She had always worked so hard. Worked hard raising three children. Worked hard on the farm with her husband. And when she developed Alzheimer's, Ruth worked incredibly hard, for many years, to cover it up.

Then Ruth had died hard—laboring to breathe, to stay alive, to keep the fire of life burning.

Muriel remembered that some of her friends, children of parents with Alzheimer's, said death was a relief. It was a release from years of suffering. Muriel wasn't so sure. It didn't seem like that for her mother. What was death really like? What would it be like for her? Was it a foe to be fought or a friend to be welcomed?

Muriel lowered the wick in the kerosene lantern and watched as the smoke curled around inside the glass globe. She walked over to the candle on the fireplace mantel. One blow. Two. A third finally snuffed the flame.

Just like Mom, thought Muriel. *Just like most of us—working hard to keep our candle burning.*

Caring for the Dying

For some loved ones, death will come quietly, quickly. For others it will come only with more struggles, more suffering. The way of death is not something we can explain or understand. We can merely wait, prepare, and pray that we can make it a little easier for our loved ones and ourselves.

When the nursing home called me about a change in my mother's condition, it was the week before Easter. I made the four-hour trip out to see her and planned to go with her to the hospital for a series of tests related to gastrointestinal bleeding she had developed. But just prior to her scheduled tests, Mom's condition deteriorated and it was soon apparent to all concerned that the primary concern was now related to her breathing.

I was faced with a decision. My mother's physician gave me the options: acute hospital care or comfort care at the nursing home with a staff well equipped to keep my mother as pain-free and comfortable as possible. I chose the latter course of action and spent the next three days (and most of the evenings and nights) sitting at her bedside, holding her hand, and assisting the nurses and aides with her personal care. When death came, it was not without a struggle, for both of us; but it came as I would have hoped it would. Mom was not alone. It was clearly evident from the tears of the nursing assistants that I was not the only "family member" who had loved her.

The following suggestions, written prior to my mother's nursing home experience and ultimate death, are ones I would still recommend, with a few additions based on my own, more personal, experience.

Caring for someone approaching the final days of life either at home or in a nursing facility is not very different from caring for any other very ill person. If your loved one is confined to a bed and needs total care for a lengthy period, your goals are to keep him or her comfortably positioned, clean, dry, and as pain-free as possible.

➤ Keep the room aired out and well lighted. Good ventilation makes breathing easier and provides a more pleasant environment for

you to work in. A dark room can be a frightening place for someone who is dying, especially someone with Alzheimer's.

➤ Because of poor circulation, your loved one may feel cold. This
will be especially noticeable in the hands and feet. Lightweight
blankets and comforters will help.

➤ Skin care is vitally important as poor circulation and inadequate
nutrition take their toll on the body's ability to nourish cells.

➤ Turn your loved one frequently, at least every two hours. Give
soothing back rubs. Pay special attention to the skin over any bony
prominences like the hips, bottom of the spine, heels, elbows,
shoulders, and even the back of the head and the ears. Consider
obtaining a water, air, or foam mattress for the bed to prevent skin
breakdown.

➤ Heels and elbows can be padded and wrapped with gauze if your
loved one thrashes against side rails. Sheepskin and foam booties
are also available.

➤ Position your loved one with extra pillows to increase comfort
and decrease pressure on legs and arms.

➤ Bowel and bladder control will diminish even more until there is
total incontinence. Keep your loved one as clean and dry as possible.
   A catheter, which may be inserted by a community-health nurse
with a physician's order, may help remove urine from the bladder.
This can easily be maintained at home, provided your loved one
is relatively still and doesn't pull it out.

➤ Keeping your loved one hydrated and nourished will become increasingly difficult. The ability to swallow may eventually be lost
altogether. In the meantime, provide favorite foods that are high
in calories.
   When swallowing becomes more difficult, offer puddings, yogurt, pureed fruits, ice cream, and sherbet. Sometimes milk

products and citrus fruit juices will increase mucus production and cause problems. If this is the case, switch to nondairy products and noncitrus juices, such as apple and cranberry. Thickeners are available for juices and can even be put in water to make swallowing easier. Home-care supply stores should be able to obtain these for you.

➤ Ice chips may be welcome if sucking can be done without danger of choking. When swallowing becomes more of a problem, moisten gauze in ice water and let your loved one suck on it. I did this with my mother; I needed to remember, however, to keep a firm grip on the gauze so she wouldn't inadvertently swallow it.

➤ Good mouth care is essential. Your loved one will probably breathe through the mouth, and the jaw will sag. The mouth can become very dry and uncomfortable as a result. Frequent liquids can help, but also consider purchasing some mouth swabs. Use them often.

➤ Placing a very light layer of petroleum jelly on lips and around nasal passages may help prevent cracking.

➤ If your loved one is bothered by an excessive amount of mucus buildup in the mouth, you may want to rent a suction machine. You can hire an in-home nurse to work this, or receive instruction from a community-health agency on its use for yourself.

➤ A sitting or semi-sitting position is best for eating and can help prevent choking. (Renting or borrowing an adjustable hospital bed will make this more practical.)

One of the best investments you can make at any time during your loved one's illness is a good nurse's aide or nursing assistant manual. Such manuals offer hundreds of additional tips on how to feed, position, bathe, toilet, and otherwise meet the physical needs of people who are ill. Titles may change from year to year; inquire through a nursing home or home-care agency about what book they use and order one through them, or from the publisher or any bookstore.

Should terminal care prove overwhelming for you, consider getting outside assistance through a local nursing agency or hospice program. The latter features professional caregivers, paraprofessionals, and volunteers who emphasize pain control and meeting the physical, emotional, and spiritual needs of patient and caregiver, in as natural an environment as possible. Medicare often reimburses some costs associated with terminal care in the home. In addition, some agencies offer sliding-fee scales based on ability to pay.

Some nursing homes also provide hospice-type care for the terminally ill during the last weeks of their life; this may be available in your area.

Emotional and Spiritual Support

"What is it about death that makes you afraid?" I once asked an elderly woman in a nursing home.

"The dying part," she replied.

"But what about the dying part?" I asked, hoping she'd be more specific.

"The part about dying alone," she said.

We can provide emotional support for loved ones simply by being with them. We can hold their hands, offer back rubs, and remind them that we love them. We can assure them they won't be abandoned. They are not alone.

We can also pray for our loved ones, asking God to ease their last days and make the transition from this life to the next an easier one. When Jesus faced his own death, he spent hours praying to God. Likewise, he expected his disciples to pray too. He needed their prayer, their emotional and spiritual support, their "being there" for him.

That is all our loved ones really ask of us. To sit and wait with them for the door of death to open.

I once led weekly Bible studies in a nursing home with a small group of Alzheimer's sufferers. Our favorite passage, and one we read frequently, was Psalm 23. It is a psalm about death. It is also a psalm about life—eternal life with God. It recognizes that death does not have to be a lonely experience. There is someone to walk through the valley of the shadow of death with us. That someone is God.

Another Bible passage I sometimes used with the group was from the book of John, chapter 14. In this account, Jesus is discussing his impending death and comforting his disciples, who are troubled and frightened. Jesus encourages them not to fear, but to trust in him. Yes, he is definitely going to die. But death will not be the end; he's coming back. He will defeat death by rising from his tomb. The disciples have no reason to fear for his death or their own.

Jesus tells his disciples that, after his resurrection, he will go to prepare a place for them in heaven. And when the disciples die, Jesus himself will usher them into the presence of God. Jesus, in fact, is the avenue from this life to the next.

That is great news. It means our candle won't go out for good but will burn brightly again on the other side of death's door. Remind your loved one of this. Remind yourself.

Brightly Burning Wicks

A number of years before my mother's death I broke my mother's cane. It happened the morning I was late for work because the aide I had hired was late. "My car broke down," she said on the phone. "I'll be there when I can."

Frustration. I was supposed to be covering for a sick coworker at the office. I had to get there as soon as possible.

My mother wasn't helping any. When I tried to get her out of bed, she resisted. When I finally got her on her feet, she decided to sit down on the floor. That's when she began striking my legs with her cane. She didn't hit me hard, but I lost control. I grabbed the cane and banged it against the floor. The cane, old and fragile, snapped in two. It lay broken on the floor beside my mother.

I felt shame and horror. My first thought was, *What if that had been Mom? Would anger or frustration ever make me treat her like that cane?*

My mother brought me back to the present. She was still sitting on the floor. But now she was laughing. I sat down beside her, put my arms around her and laughed too. I laughed until I cried.

That night I read this verse: "A bruised reed he will not break, and a dimly burning wick he will not quench" (Isaiah 42:3, RSV). That struck a nerve. At times, I felt like a bruised reed, bruised and battered in the battle against Alzheimer's.

My mother was a bruised reed too, a fragile person incapable of caring for herself or understanding what was happening. A person who needed to be cared for gently—with love, laughter, and, occasionally, tears.

But the verse in Isaiah held a promise from God. Neither of us would be broken. Neither of us had to walk through life alone. God promised to hold our hands. He would also *stay* my hand and give me patience with my mother and myself.

Later, I hauled the broken cane out of the garbage and put it in the linen closet. And now, seven years later, the broken cane rests on a shelf in another closet where I currently live, serving as a reminder for me to be gentle with those whose lives are flickering in the darkness.

Bruised reeds and dimly burning wicks. Nowhere has God promised to take us out of this world of suffering and confusion. He does promise to walk through it with us, encouraging us along the way as we care for our loved one and for ourselves. We are not alone.

Appendix A

References and Resources for Family and Professional Caregivers

The Alzheimer's Association
The national Alzheimer's Association has extensive resources for family and professional caregivers, including a quarterly newsletter with up-to-date information on all the latest research and resources. For information, support services, and to be placed on the mailing list, write or call:

The Alzheimer's Association
919 North Michigan Avenue
Suite 1000
Chicago, IL 60611-1676

Toll-free Information and Referral Line:
(800) 272-3900
Fax: (312) 335-1110

Alzheimer's Library
The Benjamin B. Green-Field National Alzheimer's Library and Resource Center located at the Alzheimer's Association headquarters in Chicago, Illinois, has developed comprehensive and annotated reading lists on a variety of specialized subjects related to dementia. These include resource lists for books, articles, journals, videos, and brochures. If material is not available through a local library or a local Alzheimer's chapter, some resources can be borrowed through

the National Library. For further information on the Library's collection or services, contact the Library at (312) 335-9602.

Some of the information available through the National Library include bibliographies and resource lists for the following:

Information for Children and Adolescents

End-Stage Issues in Alzheimer's Disease

Spirituality and Dementia Care (includes extensive resources for clergy as well as family caregivers)

Family Caregiver Stress in Dementia Care

Early-Onset Alzheimer's Disease

Nutrition and Eating Patterns of Dementia Patients

Activities for Alzheimer's Patients

Behavioral Symptoms of Alzheimer's Disease

Down Syndrome and Alzheimer's Disease

Publications

For a catalog and order form of the national Alzheimer's Association publications, including brochures, books, and videos, contact your local Alzheimer's chapter or call the toll-free Information and Referral Line: (800) 272-3900.

Examples of brochures and booklets available from the Alzheimer's Association are:

"Is It Alzheimer's? Ten Warning Signs"

"Family Guide for Alzheimer's Care in Residential Settings"

"Selecting a Nursing Home with a Dementia Care Unit"

"Ten Ways to Help an Alzheimer's Family"

"Caregiver Stress: Signs to Watch For . . . Steps to Take"

"Fact Sheet on Aluminum"

Journals

Current medical research and studies are available through these journals. You may find them at your local library, or subscribe to them yourself:

Alzheimer's Disease and Associated Disorders

American Journal of Alzheimer's Care and Related Disorders and Research

Related Organizations of Interest to Caregivers

Alzheimer's Disease Education and Referral Center (ADEAR)
PO Box 8250
Silver Spring, MD 20907-8250
(800) 438-4380
Fax: (301) 587-4352

American Association on Mental Retardation
444 North Capitol Street, NW
Suite 846
Washington, D.C. 20001-1512
(202) 387-1968

American Health Care Association
1201 L. Street NW
Washington, D.C. 20005
(202) 842-4444

Available through the AHCA is a free publication, "Thinking About a Nursing Home."

The Arc of the United States (national organization on mental retardation)
500 East Border Street, Suite 300
Arlington, TX 76010
(817) 261-6003
E-mail: thearc@metronet.com.

Available through The Arc are publications such as: "Developmental Disabilities and Alzheimer's Disease: What You Should Know," (1995, 43 pages) and "Alzheimer's Disease and People with Mental Retardation," (1995, 2 pages).

Impact AIDS, Inc.
3692 18th St.
San Francisco, CA 94110
(415) 861-3397

Available from Impact AIDS is: "Living with Dementia: A Guide for the Extended Family," a brochure specific to AIDS-related dementia.

National Down Syndrome Society
666 Broadway
New York, NY 10012
(800) 221-4602

National Home Care Association
228 7th Street, SE
Washington, D.C. 20003
(202) 547-7424

Alzheimer's Online: Internet Information
1. The Alzheimer's Association's Home Page internet address is: http://www.alz.org/
   The Home Page provides information about Alzheimer's disease, including caregiving strategies, research updates, and education and support opportunities. Also listed is contact information for more than 200 chapters nationwide. You can access it 24 hours a day. The Alzheimer's Home Page will also direct you to other organizations or freenets. An example of a freenet service available through internet is the opportunity to "talk" with other caregivers in your own local area.
2. The Alzheimer's Disease Education and Referral Center (ADEAR) of the National Institute on Aging (NIA) also has a web site offering publications and research news. Web site is: http://www.alzheimers.org/adear
   Available through ADEAR is a Progress Report, highlighting all the latest Alzheimer's research. Information specialists will also answer your questions about Alzheimer's disease. Call the

ADEAR Center at (800) 438-4380, or contact them by E-mail at: adear@alzheimers.org

3. The Down Syndrome World-Wide Web site is: www.nas.com/downsyn/

For Caregivers Concerned About Public Policy

Call the Alzheimer's Association's Public Policy Division at (202) 393-7737 for information about how to become involved in advocacy at the state and national levels.

For Nursing Home Personnel

Lisa Gwyther's book, *Care of Alzheimer's Patients: A Manual for Nursing Home Staff* (jointly published by the Alzheimer's Association and the American Health Care Association, 1985), is an excellent resource for people who work in nursing homes. All the common behaviors associated with Alzheimer's are reviewed with many practical suggestions for behavior management and activities. It can be ordered through the Alzheimer's Association.

Autopsy Information

Your local hospital, nursing home, and Alzheimer's Association chapter may be able to provide you with the necessary information needed for planning a brain autopsy. The national Alzheimer's Association Autopsy Assistance Network can also provide caregivers with helpful information regarding autopsy procedure and assistance with obtaining a confirmed diagnosis.

Specific information on donating brain tissue for research can also be obtained through the Autopsy Assistance Network. (Body organs of persons with Alzheimer's are not recommended for donation for transplant purposes, according to the Alzheimer's Association Medical and Scientific Advisory Board). Regional Autopsy Assistance Network representatives are also available around the country. Call the toll-free number or write the national Alzheimer's Association for information.

Appendix B
Other Causes of Dementia

There are a number of chronic disease processes that can produce dementia-like symptoms, and persons with these symptoms can be misdiagnosed as having Alzheimer's. In certain cases, symptoms of these other diseases can be controlled with medication and the disease process slowed. Known risk factors for some chronic disease processes may be modified.

I. Vascular Dementias

Multi-infarct dementia (MID). MID is one type of vascular dementia and the second most common cause of chronic irreversible dementia in older adults. Its cause is multiple strokes or infarcts in the brain related to an atherosclerotic process that narrows arteries feeding brain cells; when brain cells are not fed enough oxygen and nutrients because blood flow is cut off, they die. (This process is similar to what happens when someone has a heart attack and blood flow to cells in cardiac tissue is compromised). MID is often a corollary to untreated diabetes or hypertension.

Symptoms associated with MID may seem to appear suddenly, though multiple-stroke or mini-stroke activity has been occurring over a period of time. Persons with MID may experience periods of confusion and then periods called plateaus where there seems to be no perceptible change in memory or behavior; this process differs from the slow, steady, global decline associated with Alzheimer's. Persons with MID may exhibit specific local or focal neurological impairment related to specific areas of brain involvement, for example, slurred speech or muscle weakness in an arm and/or leg.

To complicate diagnosis, Alzheimer's disease and MID can coexist, and frequently do, in what is called a "mixed-dementia" that may account for fifteen to twenty percent of all existing chronic dementias.

Differentiating Alzheimer's from MID through various neuro-imaging techniques is of great importance (see pp. 36-38). Though multi-infarct dementia is not considered reversible, further stroke activity and associated dementia may be preventable as many of the risk factors for MID are known and controllable (for example, hypertension, diabetes, and vascular disease). Surgical, dietary, lifestyle, and pharmacologic interventions may be indicated.

Binswanger's disease is another vascular dementia associated with persistent, severe hypertension. Risk factors also include diabetes, cardiovascular disease, and recurrent hypotension. Advanced arteriosclerosis in the medullary arteries occurs with pathologic changes in the frontal subcortical white matter of the brain.

Symptoms of Binswanger's disease include difficulty swallowing (dysphagia) and difficulty articulating words (dysarthria). Difficulty walking, frequent falls, and urinary incontinence may also occur. Binswanger's is also plateau-like in progression. Control of associated risk factors may help slow or halt disease progression. Neuroimaging techniques are used to diagnose Binswanger's.

II. Prion-Related Dementia

Creutzfeldt-Jakob disease (CJD). CJD is a rare form of dementia believed to be caused by a transmissible prion protein. Though symptoms are similar to Alzheimer's, including memory impairment, behavior changes, and compromised coordination, Creutzfeldt-Jakob disease has a rapid progression, with death occurring within a year of diagnosis.

Symptoms may also include sudden jerking movements (myoclonus), an exaggerated startle reflex, and epileptic seizures. This disease can be diagnosed by brain autopsy following death due to unique pathologic changes in brain tissue; while living, there may be abnormal EEG readings.

III. Neurotransmitter Abnormalities

Parkinson's disease is caused by the absence of dopamine, a neurotransmitter that controls muscle activity. People with Parkinson's may also experience dementia in the late stages of this illness. In the early stages of Parkinson's, slowed or delayed thinking processes may be evident but, unlike the Alzheimer's sufferer, a person with Parkinson's, given time, will be able to remember and reason even though speech may be slower than normal. These two diseases are often confused in both early and late stages.

To confuse matters more, persons with Parkinson's may actually develop Alzheimer's, and persons with Alzheimer's may exhibit symptoms more typically characteristic of Parkinson's, for example, joint stiffness, slow movement (bradykinesia), difficulty walking or initiating movement, and sometimes complete immobility. One feature unique to Parkinson's disease and usually absent in Alzheimer's is tremors or mild to severe shaking of the hands and head.

Medication can help alleviate symptoms associated with Parkinson's, specifically the medication levodopa or L-dopa. Antidepressants are also often ordered to combat depression frequently associated with the disease.

IV. Hereditary Dementias

Huntington's disease or Huntington's Chorea. This is a hereditary disorder involving early stage cognitive changes, memory impairment, and involuntary movements (chorea) of the face and upper extremities. Depression, hallucinations, and paranoia may also occur early in the disease and progression may be a slow deterioration.

A genetic marker identified on chromosome 4 has been linked to the Huntington's gene. Pathologic changes in the brain include marked atrophy, extensive nerve cell loss, and a decrease in white matter.

Various medications may help control abnormal muscle movements, though they often lead to rigidity as a side effect. Tricyclic antidepressants are often used to combat depression.

V. Motor Neuron Abnormalities

Amyotrophic lateral sclerosis (ALS). ALS is often called "Lou Gehrig's disease" after the famous baseball player who was one of its victims. It is characterized by progressive muscle wasting and weakness, involuntary contractions of the face, tongue atrophy and difficulty speaking, and spasticity. ALS may be due to an excess of the chemical glutamate that is responsible for relaying messages between motor neurons. Too much glutamate destroys nerve cells in the brain and spinal column.

Mental and memory changes are generally not associated with this disease, unlike many other neural degenerative diseases. ALS is commonly seen in people in their late thirties and forties.

VI. White-Matter Abnormalities

Multiple-sclerosis (MS). MS is a progressive, degenerative disease with myelin sheath and conduction pathway involvement of the central nervous system. White fiber tracts connecting white matter and neurons in the brain and spinal column are usually affected. Causative explanations include viral, immunologic, and genetic factors. CT scanning may show increased density in the white matter and MS plaques. MRI and PET scanning may also be used.

As MS progresses, memory loss, impaired judgment, and an inability to problem solve and perform calculations may occur. Earlier symptoms include generalized muscle weakness, fatigue, tremors when performing activities, numbness and tingling sensations, visual disturbances, dizziness and ringing in the ears, and disturbances with bowel and bladder function.

Because symptoms are often vague and can mimic other diseases, MS often goes undiagnosed and cognitive symptoms can easily be misinterpreted for Alzheimer's disease. MS typically occurs in the twenty- to forty-year-old age range.

VII. Other Degenerative Disorders

Pick's disease (PKD). A rarer form of dementia, PKD often manifests itself in disturbances of mood and a progressive inability to speak (aphasia) that may render a person totally mute.

Disinhibitions of a sexual nature and inappropriate social behaviors and loss of social awareness are more indicative of Pick's than of traditional Alzheimer's dementia; memory loss is not as profound as in Alzheimer's disease. Behavioral disturbances may occur later in the disease that may include hyperorality or bulimia and visual agnosia or inability to interpret visual images. PKD initially affects people in their fifties and sixties.

Like Alzheimer's, Pick's disease can best be diagnosed by brain autopsy. Plaques and tangles will be present as well as "Pick bodies" in cerebral cortex, basal ganglia, and some brainstem structures. On a CT scan, severe atrophy may be present, especially in the temporal and frontal areas of the brain.

Appendix C
Medications and Research

Research and the development of new experimental drugs is ongoing and ever-changing. Clinical drug trials are being conducted at a number of sites throughout the United States. In 1995 the Reagan Institute was established, expanding the Alzheimer's Association's existing research program of biomedical research.

For fact sheets on these experimental drug studies, contact your local chapter or call the toll-free number of the Alzheimer's Association (see appendix A). The Association also has available a kit called: "From Theory to Therapy: The Development of Drugs for Alzheimer's Disease." Ordering information can be obtained.

The following is a brief summary of the latest in Alzheimer's research in the past ten years.

I. Free Radicals and Antioxidant Therapy

Researchers have long studied the beta amyloid protein that accumulates in the brains of persons with Alzheimer's disease. Recent research yields evidence that this protein also produces free radicals, or molecules, with odd numbers of electrons that in turn are known to cause cell damage or cell death. Earlier research has shown that some antioxidants, for example, vitamin E, serve to protect cells from naturally occurring free-radical damage.

Clinical trials have included the experimental medication *deprenyl*, believed to block free-radical damage, and vitamin E that may serve to neutralize the toxic effects of free radicals. Caregivers should not give their loved ones excess doses of over-the-counter vitamin E. Excess doses of any vitamin are highly toxic.

II. The Genetic Question

In 1987 researchers discovered evidence for a gene(s) on chromosome 21 related to Alzheimer's disease specifically in some families with early-onset familial Alzheimer's disease (FAD). FAD occurs in one to ten percent of all persons with Alzheimer's disease and has been known to occur in persons in their thirties. Chromosome 21 is the same chromosome associated with the occurrence of Down syndrome; abnormalities in the brain that occur in persons with Down syndrome by age forty are similar to those occurring in the Alzheimer's victim, including the characteristic plaques and tangles. Also in 1987, the gene that contains the code for the amyloid precursor protein (APP) was found on chromosome 21. APP is related to beta amyloid protein and senile plaque formation.

In 1992 the APP gene on chromosome 14 was found to contain a mutation(s) associated with some early-onset familial Alzheimer's disease cases that affected persons in their forties.

In 1993 chromosome 19 was found to have a genetic mutation more than three times as common in persons with both late-onset FAD and sporadic AD (no "known" relatives had Alzheimer's disease) than in persons without Alzheimer's disease. This gene is called apolipoprotein E (ApoE). ApoE appears to be the first biological risk factor for late-onset Alzheimer's (other than age itself).

The study of the ApoE gene is one of the most promising avenues of research. In the future there may be ways to reduce a person's risk of developing Alzheimer's, for example, by manipulating metabolism to postpone Alzheimer's, according to Duke University researchers.

III. Environmental Factors

Though to date the only established known risk factors for Alzheimer's disease are age, family history, and genetic predisposition, researchers believe some factor(s) in the environment may also play a part in the development of the disease. The study of various metals in the environment such as aluminum, mercury, and zinc is ongoing. To date the research has yielded mixed results.

Chelation therapy is sometimes advertized in popular self-help magazines as a means of ridding the body of excess aluminum or zinc. But the side effects, including hypotension, vomiting, anemia, irregular heartbeat, congestive heart failure, and kidney failure, far outweigh the proposed benefits. Caregivers should beware of fraudulent advertising and seek advice from the Alzheimer's Association or a reputable medical center before subjecting their loved one to any treatment.

Another environmental area of exploration is related to electromagnetic fields (EMFs) from power lines and other electrical equipment. A study reported in the *American Journal of Epidemiology* in September 1995 found increased likelihood of dementia in persons exposed to frequent and high levels of EMFs; this research needs to be replicated before conclusions can be reached about possible links between Alzheimer's and EMFs.

Long-term exposure to pesticides is also considered to be a possible risk factor for dementia and is under investigation.

IV. Acetylcholine Research and Related Medications

The experimental drug THA (Tacrine, or Cognex™—Parke-Davis) was first tested in 1986. The drug was designed to inhibit the breakdown of acetylcholine in the brain, a substance known to be depleted in the brains of people with Alzheimer's and believed to be associated with memory function. It has more recently been approved by the FDA as the first drug released for the treatment of mild to moderate Alzheimer's. To date it is the only FDA-approved drug treatment specifically for Alzheimer's. One side effect is liver toxicity, common to other experimental drugs. The jury is still out as to its effectiveness.

ENA 713 is another drug currently being used on an experimental basis. It inhibits the enzyme responsible for acetylcholine breakdown.

V. Mitochondria Research

Mitochondria are slender microscopic filaments. They are considered the source of energy for cells and are involved in protein synthesis and lipid or fat metabolism. Acetyl-l-carnitine naturally occurs in human cells and effects the proper functioning of mitochondria. The drug Alcar is currently being tested on an experimental basis at a number of sites in the United States in people of ages forty-five to sixty-five.

VI. Vascular Dementia Treatment

Propentofylline (HWA 285) is a drug that improves blood flow and the metabolism of energy in the brain. It has been used experimentally in some research centers across the United States.

Notes

Chapter One: Bruised Reeds and Dimly Burning Wicks

1. See the *Diagnostic and Statistical Manual of Mental Disorders*, 3rd ed., revised, (Washington, D.C.: American Psychiatric Association, Committee on Nomenclature and Statistics, 1987).

2. Statistics from the U.S. Bureau of Census, 1990; D. G. Fowles, *A Profile of Older Americans*, (Washington, D.C.: American Association of Retired Persons, 1993); The National Institute on Aging; and the Alzheimer's Association, 1994–1995.

3. Quote attributed to Dr. Lewis Thomas.

4. *The 36-Hour Day*, by Nancy Mace and Peter Rabins, is a classic in the field of dementia, (New York: Johns Hopkins University Press, Warner Books, 1992).

Chapter Two: Searching for the Truth

1. M. F. Mendez; A. R. Mastri; J. H. Sung; and W. H. Frey, "Clinically Diagnosed Alzheimer's Disease: Neuropathologic Findings in 650 Cases," *Alzheimer's Disease and Associated Disorders* 6 (1992): 35–43. Brain autopsy results on persons previously diagnosed with Alzheimer's disease showed 78 percent had been correctly diagnosed when living, suggesting clinical diagnostic criteria currently used are relatively accurate.

2. A comprehensive source book describing the various types of dementia is *Dementia: Presentations, Differential Diagnosis, and Nosology*, edited by V. Olga B. Emery and Thomas E. Oxman, (Baltimore, MD: Johns Hopkins University Press, 1995). Written for physicians and other professional caregivers, it is highly readable and includes extensive references to ongoing research that may be of interest to family caregivers needing more comprehensive information.

3. Linda Teri, "Behavioral Treatment of Depression in Patients with Dementia," *Alzheimer's Disease and Associated Disorders* 8, Suppl. 3 (1994): 66–74.

4. Two examples of mental state assessment tools are the Mini-Mental State Exam and the Blessed-Roth Dementia Scale. (M. F. Folstein; S. A. Folstein; and P. R. McHugh, "Mini Mental State: A Practical Method for Grading the Cognitive State of Patients for the Clinician," *Journal of Psychiatric Research*, 12, no. 3 (1975): 189–98; G. Blessed; B. E. Tomlinson; and M. Roth, "Blessed-Roth Dementia Scale," *Psychopharmacology Bulletin* 24, no. 4 (1988): 705–708.

5. Robert D. Terry, Robert Katzman, and Katherine L. Bick, eds. *Alzheimer's Disease* (New York: Raven Press, 1994). A book written for health-care professionals, but also an excellent source of more detailed information for family caregivers seeking medical references on the diagnostic and treatment aspects of dementia.

Chapter Three: Facing the Facts

1. Lewis Thomas, *The Medusa and the Snail* (New York: Viking Press, 1979), pp. 169–170.

2. T. Crook; R. T. Bartus; S. H. Ferris; P. Whitehouse; G. D. Cohen; and S. Gershon, "Age-Associated Memory Impairment: Proposed Diagnostic Criteria and Measures of Clinical Change-report of a National Institute of Mental Health Work Group," *Developmental Neuropsychology* 2 (1986): 26–76.

V. A. Kral, "Senescent Forgetfulness: Benign and Malignant," *Canadian Medical Association Journal* 86, no. 6 (1962): 257–60.

3. William R. Markesbery, and William D. Ehmann, "Brain Trace Elements in Alzheimer's Disease," in *Alzheimer's Disease,* edited by Terry, Katzman, and Bick (New York: Raven Press, 1994), pp. 353–367.

4. Mirian K. Aronson, ed., *Understanding Alzheimer's Disease* (New York: Charles Scribner's Sons, 1988).

Chapter Four: What's Happening Upstairs?

1. Other neurotransmitters under investigation are norepinephrine, serotonin, somatostatin, and corticotrophin-releasing factor. All are believed to be deficient in persons with Alzheimer's disease.

2. Alzheimer's disease is staged in a variety of ways in the research literature; no two people progress exactly alike.

Chapter Five: When Memory Starts to Fade

1. Naomi Feil has developed workshops and resource material on communicating with the old who are confused, focusing on their feelings. She calls her technique "Validation Therapy." See Naomi Feil, *Validation: The Feil Method* (Cleveland, OH: Edward Feil Productions, 1989).

Chapter Seven: Always on the Move

1. A volunteer walker's program was instituted by Sharon Holmberg, (R.N., Ph.D), at St. John's Nursing Home in Rochester, New York, providing a supervised hour of walking in the early evening for persons with dementia. Caregivers who have built structured walking times into their loved one's routine have commented on improved sleep and less overall restlessness.

Chapter Eight: Baffling Behaviors

1. Quote originally attributed to Janet Sawyer, Blumenthal Jewish Home, Clemmons, North Carolina.

2. Lore K. Wright, *Alzheimer's Disease and Marriage* (Newbury Park: Sage Publications, 1993), p. 7.

Chapter Nine: The Struggle for Safety

1. Recent research comparing persons diagnosed with Alzheimer's and older adults without symptoms of dementia indicates that persons with dementia show statistically significant differences in their ability to react to dangerous situations commonly encountered when driving, and to execute emergency measures to avoid accidents.

Chapter Twelve: Our Tangled Emotions

1. Granger Westberg, *Good Grief* (Philadelphia: Fortress Press, 1971), p. 20.

2. J. C. S. Breitner, "Clinical Genetics and Genetic Counseling in Alzheimer's Disease," *Annals of Internal Medicine* 115, no. 8 (1991): 601–606.

3. C. Oliver and A. J. Holland, "Down Syndrome and Alzheimer's Disease: A Review," *Psychological Medicine* 16 (1986): 307–322.

4. Karl Menninger, *Whatever Became of Sin?* (New York: Hawthorn Books, 1973), pp. 1–2.

5. Illustration from Jeff Smith, *The Frugal Gourmet Cooks with Wine* (New York: William Morrow and Company, 1986), pp. 75–76.

Chapter Thirteen: Hot But Not Burned Up

1. Hugh Silvester, *Arguing with God* (Downers Grove: InterVarsity Press, 1972).

2. C. S. Lewis, *A Grief Observed* (New York: Bantam Books, 1976), pp. 34–35.

3. Bernard Mobbs, *Our Rebel Emotions* (New York: Seabury Press, 1970).

4. Christopher Fitzsimons Allison, *Guilt, Anger, and God* (New York: Seabury Press, 1972).

5. Quote attributed to Martin Luther in Thomas McCormick and Sharon Fish, *Meditation: A Practical Guide to a Spiritual Discipline* (Downers Grove: InterVarsity Press, 1983), p. 10.

Chapter Fourteen: Joy in the Mourning

1. Granger Westberg, *Good Grief*, p. 30.

2. Westberg, p. 33.

3. Robert Davis, *My Journey into Alzheimer's Disease: A Story of Hope* (Wheaton: Tyndale House, 1989), p. 114.

4. Elisabeth Elliot, *Loneliness* (Nashville: Oliver Nelson, 1988).
5. Davis, *My Journey into Alzheimer's Disease*, p. 86.
6. Ibid., p. 120.

Chapter Fifteen: The Difficult Decisions

1. Nancy L. Mace and Peter V. Rabins, *The 36-Hour Day* (New York: Johns Hopkins University Press, Warner Books Edition, 1992), p. 326.

Index